Introduction to Genetic Toxicology

Introduction to Genetic Toxicology

Written and translated by
J. Moutschen
Laboratoire de Génétique
Université de Liège
Belgium

With a preface by
Lars Ehrenberg
Wallenberg Laboratory
University of Stockholm
Sweden

A Wiley–Interscience Publication

JOHN WILEY & SONS
Chichester · New York · Brisbane · Toronto · Singapore

First published under the title *Introduction à la Toxicologie Génétique* by Masson, Paris, 1979

Library of Congress Cataloguing in Publication Data:

Moutschen, Jean.
Introduction to genetic toxicology.

'A Wiley–Interscience publication.'
Translation of: Introduction à la toxicologie génétique.
Bibliography: p.
Includes index.
1. Chemical mutagenesis. 2. Genetic toxicology.
I. Title. [DNLM: 1. Mutagens. 2. Mutation—drug effects.
QH465.C5 M924i]
QH465.C5M6813 1984 575.2'92 84–11868
ISBN 0 471 90143 1

British Library Cataloguing in Publication Data:

Moutschen, J.
Introduction to genetic toxicology.
1. Chemical mutagenesis 2. Toxicology
I. Title II. Introduction à la toxicologie génétique. *English*
575.2'92 QH465.C5

ISBN 0 471 90143 1

Typeset by Inforum Ltd, Portsmouth
Printed in Great Britain by Page Bros., (Norwich) Ltd.

This book is dedicated
to my wife

Contents

Preface

Introduction to Genetic Toxicology is a survey of the problems posed in environmental toxicology, considered from a genetic point of view. It is an intricate matter in a rapidly growing field. However, since the author tries to impart his own knowledge, sprinkled with original ideas about various subjects, the reading becomes easy and attractive, being intended for students as well as for persons such as administrators or politicians who are concerned with environmental problems. A choice of judiciously selected references allows the reader who wishes to go deeper into specific scientific details to go back to the sources.

This is the reason why, after reading through the book, I am pleased to endorse the wish of Dr. Moutschen in making some personal statements derived from the text about the risks of environmental mutagens for man.

The original French issue of this monograph was provided with two prefaces, the first by Dr. A. Lafontaine, then Director of the Institute of Hygiene and Epidemiology, Brussels, and the second by myself. Having agreed to provide the present English version of the book with a translation of my preface, I feel it pertinent also to consider a few of Dr. Lafontaine's important and elegantly formulated viewpoints.

With regard to the risks run by man (and his compatriots in the animal and plant kingdoms), Dr. Lafontaine remarks that, whereas we see today a rapid progress of the evaluation of threats concerned with carcinogenesis and also teratogenesis, there has been a much slower development of sensitive methods for systematic studies of heritable damage with regard to consequences to the future chances of today's species.

This state of affairs certainly reflects the fact that, as far as man is concerned, it is easier to establish cause–effect relationships for somatic than for heritable consequences of damage to the genetic material of cells. But the level of knowledge in a scientific field is always related to priorities made in the definition of the 'research front', and these priorities are coupled to sources of funds which are in their turn closely correlated with the values of politicians and of the opinions supporting their power. And politicians are generally operating on a short-term perspective — one or two election periods. As far as health hazards are concerned, this short-term perspective of politicians coincides with the electors' egotistic fear of cancer and other diseases in their own generation, including the fear of begetting malformed children. In contrast, it is difficult to arouse a similar interest in the possibility that what we call technological progress may lead to an impairment of the health of our descendants in a remote future.

Partly due to imperfect epidemiological techniques and lack of adequate 'translation factors' from laboratory organisms to man, knowledge of the magnitude of such heritable damage is in fact so incomplete that we are unable to rule out the possibility of a genetic catastrophe. And those future citizens of the world, who will maybe accuse twentieth-century generations by saying, 'See what they did to us!', are left unheard in the setting of today's priorities.

In particular, the egotistic favouring of the interests of our generation may have severe consequences for future man when, at periods of economic crisis, first priority is given to productivity and security of employment, risks of late health effects becoming a matter of secondary importance.

Considering other species, the future of man, in his interplay with the environment, is still more threatened by the now ongoing loss of variation (i.e. of genetic information developed during multimillion-year-long evolution) caused by technological progress in a much broader sense than activities leading to the emission of mutagens.

The author discusses in a stimulating way various efforts to quantify risks of heritable harm. In this context he does not forget to touch upon the ethical problems involved in decisions about the permissibility of exposures and of the danger involved in man's intervention with his own species.

Being a valuable introduction, for students of science as well as for laymen, to known and desirable facts about the interaction of environmental factors with the genetic material of the species, Dr. Moutschen's monograph will at the same time create a sound background of taking responsibility in the difficult problems concerned.

LARS EHRENBERG

Introduction

During the last decades, alarming ideas arose because of the increased presence in our environment of new chemicals, and also from the appraisal of new techniques. Already in 1957, Ehrenberg and Gustafsson (see Ehrenberg and Gustafsson, 1970) drew the attention of the Swedish medical authorities to the urgent necessity to investigate in detail the potential mutagenic and carcinogenic effects of several chemicals to provide against these hazards.

In 1968, Epstein (cited by Sanders, 1969) stated: 'I believe the risks from mutagenicity may well transcend those of cancer. It is incomprehensible to me that some 10 to 20 years after radiation hazards have been at least partially assessed, we have no firm knowledge of the mutagenic hazards of chemicals in the human environment.'

What is responsible for this situation? First, it should be pointed out that people have been long to realize the occurrence of such hazards. Also the information in this field has for a long time been practically non-existent. Finally, it should be remembered that the initial aim of the geneticists in the field of mutagenesis was to use the most powerful mutagens for plant and animal improvements or as a tool for genetic analysis (Auerbach, 1976, in Gen. Refs.).

Beside this somewhat positive aspect of mutagenesis, it must be recognized at once that mutagens can also exert deleterious effects in man, by inducing hereditary diseases. After a long maturation period the idea was fully formulated that mutagens were actually increasingly present in the environment, and that it was urgent to prevent noxious effects.

Scientific societies progressively evolved in several countries. First, Hollaender created the Environmental Mutagen Society in the USA. Similar societies, efficiently working together, have evolved in Europe, Japan and India. These societies are not confined to geneticists but also include toxicologists, hygienists, ecologists, manufacturers and physicians; namely, all persons interested in one way or another in the future of man and in the preservation of the environment. Since their creation, these societies have regularly organized international meetings as well as workshops in conjunction with industry and the medical authorities of various countries. Local sections of these societies are now active. Beyond the basic problems, one task is to investigate the specific problems of each country.

In 1969, in the United States scientists were chiefly interested in mutations produced by pesticides, for which a committee of 'Health Education and Welfare' was created. In 1972, a conference on the human environment was held in Stockholm, a part of which, following the tradition of this country, aimed to evaluate genetic hazards (Ramel, 1973). In 1973, the first international conference on environmental mutagens was held in Asilomar in California, a second in Edinburgh in 1977, and the last in Japan in 1981. This field is still expanding. Even the legal aspects of the problems are currently being explored. In the United States, laws have been proposed by congressmen to extend the present legislation to chemical mutagens (Public Law 94–469, 11th October, 1976, 94th Congress 1978) and also more recently in the EEC (Loprieno, 1983). Mutagenicity is now identified as a hazard for public health.

Before coming to the core of the matter, we should first explain what is meant by genetic toxicology.

The potential toxicity of chemicals occurring in the environment is a familiar concept. In everyday life, when the parameters are generally well defined, it is almost routine work. If the toxicity of a chemical is to be evaluated, it is first given to a number of animals, generally a mammal, then after a suitably selected time, the number of survivors is counted. The dose of the chemical that kills half the animals treated within a given time is called the lethal dose 50% or LD_{50}*. After fixing this parameter, and in some cases after comparing the sensitivity of different species, it is required to describe the effects of the chemicals by investigating in detail the functional modifications of the organism and of each organ in particular, i.e. the physiopathological and anatomopathological reactions.

Finally, the last step should attempt to elucidate the mechanism of action at the molecular level. For pharmaceuticals, toxicological data selected from the indexes of pharmacology allow the doses required to be ascribed and the toxicity defined.

Results from epidemiological investigations of industrial pollutants allow confidence limits to be fixed and adequate action to be taken. Except in very special cases, methods used in classical toxicology take little or no account of the so-called long-term effects. These effects are essentially of three kinds:

First, substances absorbed at doses considered as showing little toxicity on the basis of classical criteria can act preferentially on the embryo at specific stages of its development, and therefore induce an anomaly resulting in a monstrosity. This is the *teratogenic* effect.

Independently from this effect, small amounts of various substances that by

* It is sometimes justified to define a dose which kills 37% of treated organisms (or LD_{37}) for agents which act by a one-hit mechanism. In this case, the proportion of survivors $A/A_\circ = e^{-aD}$ where a is the probability of hitting the target and D the dose. Thus, when $\alpha D = 1$, $A/A_\circ = e^{-1} = 0.37$.

themselves do not produce detectable toxic effects can eventually result in a malignant tumour. This is the *carcinogenic* effect.

Finally, independently from any teratogenic or carcinogenic activity, and in the longer term, various substances can, at concentrations sometimes extraordinarily small, irreversibly damage the genetic system of an organism producing effects that will only appear in further generations. This is the *mutagenic* effect.

The present handbook will deal almost exclusively with this latter aspect of toxicity.

Numerous common points exist between carcinogenesis and mutagenesis; the majority of physical and chemical agents that show mutagenicity also show carcinogenicity. It is therefore not surprising that in most treatises carcinogenicity is referred to alongside mutagenicity. This is derived from the old concept that cancers arise from somatic mutations (Bauer, 1928; Boveri, 1929, in Gen. Refs.). Nowadays, carcinogenic processes are thought to be far more complicated than a single mutation, however important that might be (Berenblum in Sutton and Harris, 1972, in Gen. Refs.) We think that, since we lack evidence about the etiological similarity of the two processes, the study of the mutagenic properties of an agent should in many respects be separate from the study of its carcinogenic effects, though these latter could in some ways serve as pilot experiments designed to evaluate mutagenic effects for the very reason that they can be detected in the exposed generation (Butterworth and Golberg, 1979, in Gen. Refs.) Cancerology — as also teratology — developed its own methods quite distinct from the genetic methodology. This is why we are excluding carcinogenic and teratogenic effects from the present handbook, without underestimating their enormous importance. We should mention, however, that during the last decade some enthusiastic ideas have emerged, attempting to link the two fields of mutagenesis and carcinogenesis despite the many question marks. It is in fact a biased approach to the problem which arose from the emergency of requiring to test thousands of substances within a short time. For this purpose, short-term tests were designed. Some carcinogenic substances were tested for mutagenicity and actually found to show positive effects in lower organisms. Therefore, if we could demonstrate that all carcinogenic substances in mammals and possibly in man have a mutagenic effect in microbes, would it not be possible that mutagenicity testing in short-term tests detects potential carcinogenicity in mammals?

Now, it must be stated that this assertion is based on no more than a correlation. It means that when we state that a carcinogenic substance for man is also mutagenic in bacteria, it has to have been previously proved by cancer methodology that it was actually carcinogenic after long-term tests in mammals. This correlation between mutagenicity and carcinogenicity can only be made at this cost. It has been found for hundreds of substances, but not for all. Therefore, if we assume that there are still classes of substances, untested in mammals, which give false results in bacteria, this makes the correlation questionable. To see how far it is possible to pursue this line of research, and also to develop new methods to correlate mutagenicity and carcinogenicity, international organisms evolved for this very purpose. One of them is the International Commission for Protection against Environmental Mutagens and Carcinogens founded in 1976 (Sobels, 1977; summary of the first five years in Sobels and Delehanty, 1982). They specialize in the field, and the objective is not only to critically evaluate the body of data presently available from which priorities for future research can be derived, but also to make recommendations for future guidelines and regulations. There are also national organizations such as the Gene-Tox programme in the United States which are investigating such problems.

After these preliminary considerations, we are now in a position to define genetic toxicology and to place it in its context.

> *'Genetic Toxicology is the systematic investigation of the effects that all physical and chemical agents present in our environment can exert on the genetic system of man as well as of their remote genetic consequences for the future of the species.'*

In the same way as traditional toxicology, its first aim is to describe the outcome produced by toxic substances in various organisms, but only from the genetic standpoint, and to draw conclusions that can be extrapolated to man. The next aim is to investigate the mechanisms of action of the substances and, on the basis of this knowledge, to evaluate the risks for man. On the other hand, genetic toxicology takes its methods only from genetics, in such a way that some researchers have called it toxicological genetics, attempting to stress the methodological aspects. We think this name is less justified than genetic toxicology, for it should be preferable to give more importance to the aims rather than to the means to reach them. The dichotomy exists, however.

Therefore, the first part of this book deals more specifically with genetic methods applicable to genetic toxicology. As a rule, these models allow all kinds of mutations to be detected and their frequency to be assessed. However, we must emphasize that the concept of genetic toxicology largely overlaps the concept of mutations and of the risk of these mutations for man. In fact, some agents can modify the population structure considerably without necessarily increasing the mutation rate, especially by modification of the recombination frequencies or by selection processes. These effects, at least as important as mutations, are much less known, however, and are going to be investigated in the future.

Furthermore, genetic toxicology not only comprises the systematic investigation of all environmental agents which can, one way or another, modify the structure of a population — the subject of the second part of this book — but also includes investigation of all regulatory processes which tend to counteract the action of these agents, and, from a prophylactic or hygienic standpoint, the study of the consequences derived from the knowledge of the genetic risks.

Before approaching the study of the genetic effects of physical and chemical agents present in the environment, we emphasize two points: first, it is obvious that the knowledge of toxic molecules has taken advantage of the spectacular progress in chemical technology. Second, in contrast, our knowledge of some genetic mechanisms especially in man has yet to be improved.

In this context, the molecular mechanisms leading to the various kinds of mutations or determining crossing-over with a somewhat mathematical precision are still poorly understood. If we consider that all the principles required to approach the study of human inheritance successfully were established at the beginning of this century, it appears that opposed ideas only could have hampered the advances in the field. These ideas possibly originated from sociocultural and political influences, i.e. from deep interactions between genetics and eugenics.

Having resolved the conflicting situation arising from divergent ideologies, human genetics is now ready to stride ahead — the gates of the future are wide open.

Acknowledgements

The author wishes to acknowledge with gratitude the encouragement and helpful attitude of the Belgian medical authorities, who clearly understand the importance of the task to be accomplished in genetic toxicology. He is most grateful to Prof. A. Lafontaine (Institute of Epidemiology and Hygiene, Brussels), who read the entire manuscript and offered helpful suggestions. He is particularly indebted to Prof. L. Ehrenberg (Wallenberg Laboratory, University of Stockholm) for valuable constructive criticisms, and also for his long-lasting and fruitful collaboration in the field. To his dear coworkers — Drs. M. Moutschen-Dahmen, N. Degraeve and J. Gilot-Delhalle (University of Liège) — he expresses his gratitude for many valuable discussions and also for their personal contributions to several topics. He offers his grateful thanks to Drs. A. Colizzi and N. Fontignie-Houbrechts who significantly contributed by working out several techniques in mammalian genetics.

Many thanks are due to Mrs. R. Verdbois-Léonard who prepared the typescript.

We are indebted for a number of the figures presented in this work, to Drs. C. Calberg-Bacq, and E. Delhalle and to M.-C. Chollet (University of Liège), to Dr. A. Sparrow (Brookhaven National Laboratory, USA), Dr. E. Chu (University of Michigan, Ann Arbor, USA), Dr. W. Nichols (Institute for Medical Research, Camden, USA), Dr. A. Malashenko (Laboratory for Experimental Biological Models, Moscow, USSR) and Dr. A. Léonard (Centre d'Energie Nucléaire, Mol, Belgium).

Finally, he thanks Prof. J. Salmon (University of Liège) for valuable suggestions in immunology.

Chapter 1

Methodology for Detecting Mutations at the Molecular and Cellular Levels

It is essential to be able to control the techniques that allow the risks of mutagenic agents found in the environment or liable to be generated therein to be assessed as precisely as possible.

Animals or plants used for this purpose are numerous, and it is not always easy to evaluate the real importance for man of the sometimes contradictory results obtained with the tests at present available. Originally, genetic technology, although elaborate, was not intended to detect mutagens in the environment. The majority of methods in mutagenesis were developed to measure the effects of physical and chemical agents well known for their high mutagenic efficiency, and not to check the risks of substances of generally weak activity compared with major mutagens.

As a whole, the tests can be separated into four groups. Some researchers consider that knowledge of the reactions of toxic compounds at the level of DNA molecules can provide sufficient information to suggest caution against potential mutagenicity (group I). Other researchers believe that an easier way to solve the problem is to use micro-organisms rather than more complicated higher organisms, arguing that this will increase the resolving power, thus the sensitivity, of the test. In micro-organisms, biochemical mutants are generally thought to be more convenient for this purpose compared with more complex morphological mutants (group II). Other researchers are trying to improve methods to reveal the damage directly induced by mutagenic agents at the chromosomal level (group III). Finally, other researchers prefer a less rapid but more fundamental genetic approach, that of observing the effects in the progeny of treated organisms (group IV). A set of test systems available is briefly summarized below.

Classification of tests available

Group I: Tests designed to detect lesions at the molecular level

a. In DNA of various origins – microsomal fraction added or not

   Unscheduled DNA synthesis

b. In proteins, e.g. haemoglobin

Group II: Tests designed to detect mutations at the cellular level

A. Direct

a. Lower organisms

Phages

Bacteria: *Escherichia coli*, *Salmonella typhimurium, etc.*

Yeasts: *Saccharomyces cerevisiae*, *Schizosaccharomyces pombe*

Fungi: *Neurospora crassa* and other species, *Aspergillus nidulans*, various species of *Penicillium*, *Sordaria brevicollis*

Protozoa: Paramecium aurelia, Tetrahymena piriforme, etc.

b. Higher organisms

Plants: Maize (*waxy* mutants in pollen cells)
Barley (*waxy* mutants in pollen cells)
Tradescantia (mutations in stamen hairs)

Mammals: Rabbit (*in vitro* cultured cells)
Syrian hamster (*in vitro* cultured cells)
Chinese hamster (*in vitro* cultured cells)
Mouse (*in vitro* cultured cells, spot test)
Man (*in vitro* cultured cells, *in vivo* immunological detection – blood and sperm)

B. Indirect

Host-mediated assays

Rabbit: *Salmonella typhimurium*, *Neurospora crassa*

Mouse: *Salmonella typhimurium, Neurospora crassa, Schizosaccharomyces pombe*

Rat: *Salmonella typhimurium*, *Neurospora crassa*

Hamster: *Salmonella typhimurium*

Group III: Tests designed to estimate the induced chromosome damage (clastogenic effect)

A. *In vitro*

a. Plants: *Tradescantia* (pollen grains)
Trillium (pollen grains)
Carrot, *Nicotiana*, etc. (various diploid tissue cultures)

b. Animals: Numerous cell strains of rabbit, Syrian and Chinese hamsters, rat, mouse and man (including malignant tissues)

B. *In vivo*

a. Plants: Barley (root tips)
Onion (root tips)
Broad bean (root tips)
Tradescantia (pollen grains, pollen mother cells, root tips)
Trillium (pollen grains, pollen mother cells)

b. Animals: Mouse, rat, hamster (spermatogenesis, bone marrow)

Group IV: Mutagenicity testing at the level of the whole organism

a. Plants: Barley (chlorophyll mutants, induced sterility)
Maize (chlorophyll mutants, *yg2* test)
Arabidopsis thaliana (chlorophyll mutants)
Wheat (various mutants)
Pea (various mutants)

b. Animals: *Drosophila* (recessive visible and lethal sex-linked mutants, *ClB*, *Muller-5, B In sc y, facl*
Habrobracon (recessive visible lethal autosomic mutations)
Silk worm (induced mutation in oocytes)
Mouse: specific-locus mutation test, dominant lethal mutation assays, chromosomal non-disjunction, sex-linked recessive (visible and lethal) mutations, heritable translocations (hemisterility).

These methods have been described in detail in several textbooks (Burdette, 1962, 1963a, b; Fishbein *et al.*, 1970; Vogel and Röhrborn, 1970; Hollaender, 1971a, b, 1973, 1976; Hollaender and de Serres, 1978; de Serres and Hollaender, 1980, 1982; Kilbey *et al.*, 1977, and 1984, in Gen. Refs.) In Chapters 1 and 2 only some chief principles are indicated, followed by a critical discussion in Chapter 3.

Group I

Among procedures that aim to detect chemical alterations of DNA after reaction with a mutagenic agent, Marmur's (1961) method has long been used in several laboratories. It is based on the use of the transforming factor. This factor is extracted from a wild type bacterium, then treated with the mutagenic agent for a short time. After elimination of the mutagenic agent, the transforming factor is incubated with bacterial cells of a tryptophan-dependent strain; this strain is normally unable to grow on a medium not supplemented with this amino acid. A mutation of the transforming factor in the donor DNA, located near the *trp* (tryptophan) region, will transform the bacteria so that not only will they be able to grow on this tryptophanless medium, but they will also accumulate a fluorescent precursor allowing an easy and rapid count of the mutant colonies, and hence the estimation of mutagenic events induced in the donor DNA.

Treatment with the so-called microsomal fraction has been much used with a large variety of test systems not only DNA. After suitable extraction of the microsomal fraction from a tissue or a whole organ (e.g. liver, testicle or even plant organs), homogenization and centrifugation at 9000 *g* (S 9), the potential mutagen is treated with this extract for a certain time and then transferred to the test system. This treatment is designed to check how the substance is detoxified by the active fraction of the organ or, conversely, to check if a normally non-mutagenic substance (i.e. a promutagen) can be transformed into a real mutagen (Montesano and Magee, 1970; Ames *et al.*, 1973) (Chapters 8 and 10). Human cells are also used for metabolic activation of chemicals.

More recently, the demonstration of induced DNA lesions made this molecule a valuable tool for detecting potential mutagens. It can be assessed by measuring strand breakage (Kohn and Grimek-Ewig, 1973; Lee and Zbinden, 1979) or covalent binding of the chemical with DNA (Brookes and Lawley, 1964; Lutz, 1979).

There is also another possibility for indirect measurement of the damage based on the study of excision-repair processes, namely unscheduled DNA synthesis. It can be performed *in vitro,* but it is desirable to confirm the results with *in vivo* experiments. Maturation stages of the seminiferous tubules of mouse (Sega, 1974; Sega *et al.*, 1976) or rabbit (Zbinden, 1980) are selected. After administering the test substance, generally intraperitoneally, labelled thymidine (often with tritium) is injected as a precursor of DNA synthesis. Radioactive spermatozoa are collected at regular intervals, either by sacrificing the animal (mouse) or collecting sperm (rabbit). The radioactivity is accurately measured by liquid spectrometry or by autoradiography. This has become an important test which takes into account the metabolic fate of the tested substances and yields information about testicular barriers.

Another method for detecting genotoxic agents at the molecular level has been developed more recently (review in Ehrenberg and Osterman-Golkar, 1980) and is rapidly being improved. It is based on the fact that most genotoxic compounds react as electrophilic agents with well-known nucleophilic centres of macromolecules such as DNA or proteins. Thus the reactivity of a compound for a specific centre of a macromolecule (e.g. histidine or cysteine of haemoglobin) can be accurately measured. This is especially true for alkylation reactions for which this test has been developed, allowing sensitive dosimetric comparisons between the genotoxicity of various agents. Not without interest is the fact that this method can also be used for *in vitro* experimental studies as a screening technique or for *in vivo* epidemiological studies for monitoring populations (details in Chapter 9).

Group II

Tests designed to detect mutations directly involve a large number of organisms ranging from the most simple phages to the most complex mammals.

Tests on lower organisms are sometimes based on morphological mutations such as those affecting rII of phage T4, the ability of phages to lyse sensitive strains of *Escherichia coli,* variations of bacterial colonies from *S* (smooth) to *R* (rough), etc. These tests are in some ways biased. This is the reason why more accurate biochemical mutations are generally preferred: Among them, the so-called nutritional (auxotrophic) mutants have been preferred; they can be forward or reverse (back mutations).

In the first case, organisms treated with a mutagenic agent are plated on a complete medium, i.e. a medium containing all the nutritional factors (sugars, amino acids, vitamins, etc.) required for normal growth of the organism. Colonies are replicated on several media, each lacking an essential factor present in the complete medium. When a bacterium is mutant for a specific factor, it cannot grow on medium lacking this factor, and the specific requirement can be easily identified. This procedure is time-consuming. To circumvent this difficulty, simplifications have been introduced: first, by introducing the 'replica test' as described by Lederberg and Lederberg (1952; see Lederberg, 1960) and frequently used since (Fig. 1).

This technique allows numerous colonies to be transferred onto a great variety of media. The use of mutants that accumulate a fluorescent or coloured precursor allows the easy detection of colonies. Reverse mutations are sometimes preferred to forward mutations since they can be more rapidly and efficiently detected. In this case, a mutant unable to grow normally on a medium not supplemented with a definite metabolite is used. Only cells which have recovered the altered genic function can form colonies on this starved medium. This method is more specific than the previous one, but involves a smaller spectrum of mutations. It has been used mainly with the following organisms: *Salmonella typhimurium, Escherichia coli, Neurospora crassa* (*ade 3A* and *ade 3B*), *Saccharomyces cerevisiae, Schizosaccharomyces pombe* and *Aspergillus nidulans* (Fig. 2). (For a review of the numerous works on mutagenesis of such organisms, see Hollaender, 1971a, b.)

A bacterial test that has become quite popular during the last decade is the

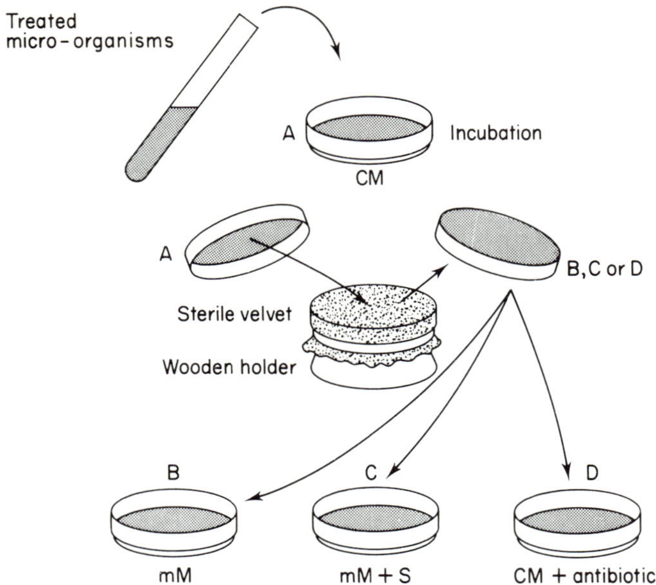

FIG. 1. Lederberg's replica test in lower organisms (bacteria, yeasts, algae). The test-tube contains the micro-organisms treated with the substance being tested for potential mutagenicity. After treatment the micro-organisms are plated on Petri dishes containing the complete medium, then incubated (dish A).
Dish A is gently pressed on a piece of sterile velvet maintained on a wooden holder. Surface colonies stick to the velvet. Dishes B, C and D containing different media according to the type of mutant investigated.
Dish A: CM = complete medium.
Dish B: mM = minimum medium.
Dish C: mM + S = minimum medium supplemented with a nutrient necessary for the growth of the micro-organism being investigated (sugar, vitamin, amino acid) to detect auxotrophic mutants.
Dish D: CM + antibiotic = complete medium supplemented with antibiotic to detect resistant mutants. (Details in the text.)

Ames test (Ames *et al.*, 1975). This test measures reverse mutations in a series of histidine-requiring auxotrophic strains of *Salmonella typhimurium* (mainly TA-1535, TA-1537, TA-1538, TA-98 and TA-100) properly selected and standardized to ensure good reproducibility. It allows both base substitutions and frameshift mutations to be detected, thanks to the presence of appropriate genetic markers. The protocol of this test was carefully worked out in all respects: the strains of bacteria, the number of concentrations of the potential mutagen tested, the solvents, the way to make the controls, and also the activation system after adding microsomal enzymes (see above). Thousands of substances have been investigated with this test system which can now be considered routine. This test was also devised to correlate the carcinogenicity and mutagenicity of the investigated compounds (McCann *et al.*, 1975). This correlation is established by observing positive mutagenic effects in bacteria and cancer induction in mammals, generally rodents. For hundreds of subst-

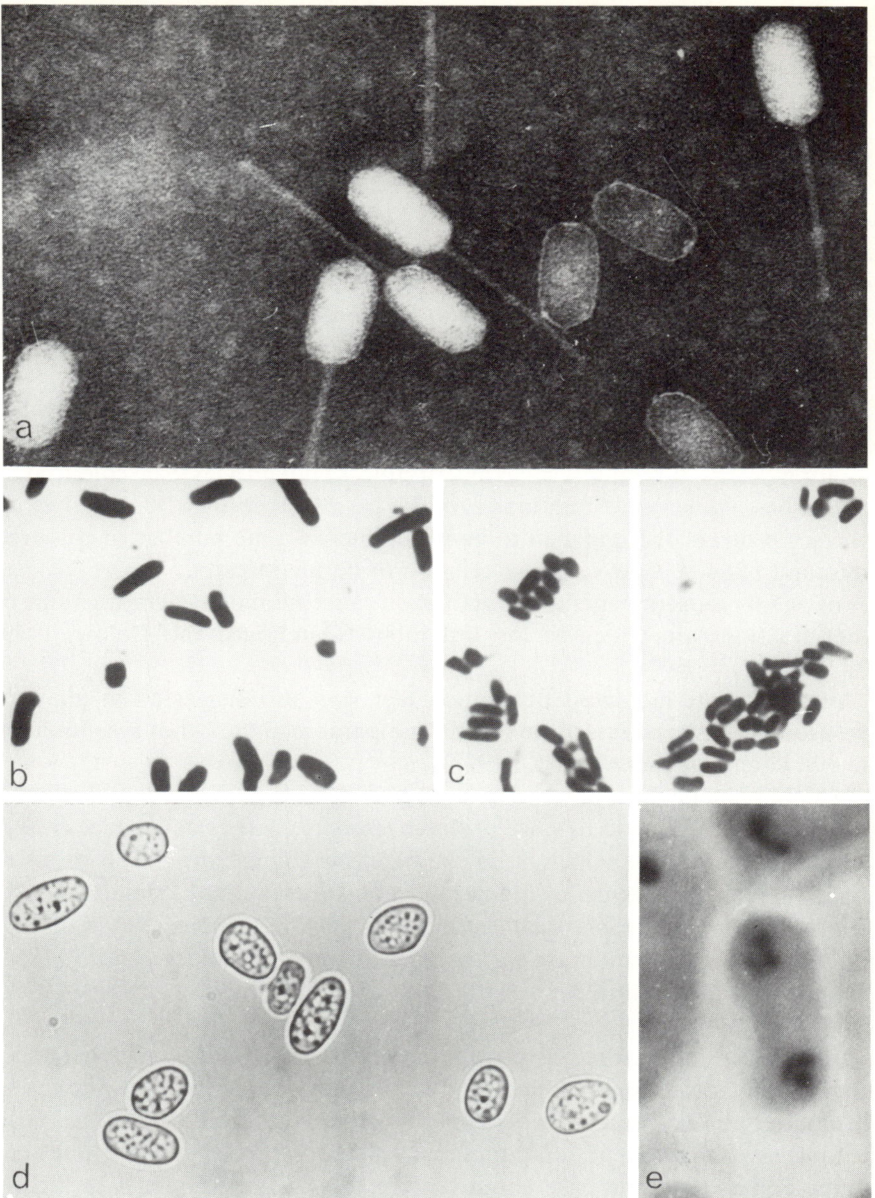

Fig. 2. Examples of micro-organisms in current use for mutagenicity testing. a. Electron micrograph of a bacterial virus (bacteriophage R_2 infectious for *Streptomyces*). Negative contrast with phosphotungstate. Complete particles have an elongated polyhedric head (100 nm × 50 nm) and a rigid tail (170 nm long). (Picture by courtesy of Dr. C.-M. Calberg-Bacq, Université de Liège, Laboratoire de Microbiologie Générale et médicale). b. Smear of *Escherichia coli* stained with Giemsa and observed with a photomicroscope (× 1200). c. Smear of *Salmonella typhimurium* stained with Giemsa and observed with a photomicroscope (× 1200). d. *Schizosaccharomyces pombe* after cytological fixation. Observation by phase microscopy (× 600). e. cell division of *Schizosaccharomyces pombe* stained with Giemsa (× 1200). (Pictures b–e: Dr. J. Moutschen).

ances tested, this correlation is said to be good, but for some classes of substances, the results are still controversial (review in Mohn, 1981).

Resistance of bacteria to phages and antibiotics is also commonly proposed as a criterion of mutagenicity (Lederberg and Lederberg, 1952).

Another test for the detection of mutations in bacteria is the fluctuation test, which was first designed by Luria and Delbrück (1943) to study bacterial variation. Subsequently, it was transformed into a mutation test in a variety of genetic systems, and then into a screening test (review in Bridges, 1980). The test can be performed with Ames *Salmonella* strains or *E. coli WP 2 trp* and related strains, yeasts (Parry, 1977) and mouse lymphoma cells (Cole *et al.*, 1976).

Bacteria under test are added to media in test tubes containing traces of the required amino acid adjusted to restrict the level of residual growth. If a mutation occurs, it ferments sugar and produces enough acid to be coloured by an acid-base indicator. Mutations can also be indicated by turbidity. Higher concentrations of the mutagen to be tested increase the number of coloured tubes and allow a dose–response relation to be investigated.

For agents requiring metabolic activation, microsomal rat liver fractions or other fractions are added to the test tubes (Gatehouse and Delow, 1979; Hubbard *et al.*, 1980).

An hepatocyte-mediated fluctuation test was also suggested in place of microsomal enzymes. It is more closely comparable to the conditions found in the whole animal (Green *et al.*, 1977).

In higher plants, the most commonly tested cells are pollen grains. A specific mutation controls the occurrence of starch (*starchy: Wx*) or its absence (*waxy: wx*). The starch in the pollen grain can be easily stained with a few drops of Lugol's iodine (a mixture of iodine and potassium iodide). Simultaneously described in maize by Brink and MacGillivray (1924), Demerec (1924) and Longley (1924), this mutation was used in this test system by Nelson (1957, 1968). The same mutation was efficiently used in barley by Erikson (1962, 1969).

As in lower organisms, it is possible to check direct mutations by staining starch of mutants in a population of pollen, or reverse mutations by counting the number of *waxy* mutants in a population of *starchy* pollen grains (Fig. 3). In the first case, the frequency of spontaneous mutations in barley was about 1 per million and in the latter case about 1 per 100 000. The frequency is slightly higher in maize (Ehrenberg and Eriksson, 1966). This test system has the advantage of being easily performed on large cell populations (10^7 cells without too much work) which increases the sensitivity. This method has been so much improved that in an 8-hour day one worker can prepare the slides and screen 1 million pollen grains (Rosichan *et al.*, 1981).

Such test systems with pollen allow all mutations to be expressed due to the haploid state of the pollen cells, no gene being masked. Since each pollen grain is in fact the equivalent of a whole organism, this test could as well be classified in group IV. However, since it has more affinity with micro-organism tests, it is

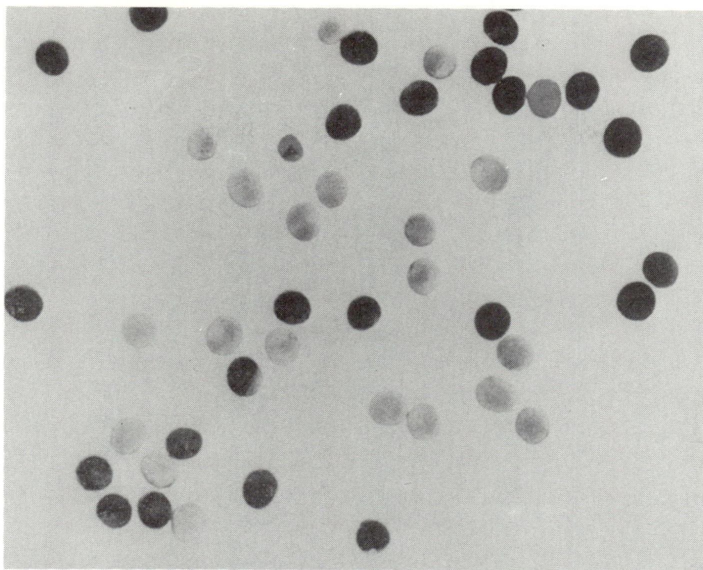

FIG. 3. Pollen grains of maize heterozygous for the gene *waxy* (*wx*). After staining with Lugol's mixture, only *starchy* (*Wx*) grains are stained (after Demerec)

preferable to classify it under the present heading.

The estimation of the frequency of anthocyanic mutants in *Tradescantia* staminal hairs (a test developed by Sparrow *et al*; see Ichikawa and Sparrow, 1968) rests on the same criteria as pollen mutants (Fig. 4). Staminal hairs are directly treated with the mutagenic agent to be tested, and the somatic effects are scored at the following cell division or even later. The loss of the reproductive capability as well as morphological modifications can be checked (Ichikawa *et al.*, 1969; Underbrink *et al.*, 1973). Mainly the effects of very low doses of ionizing radiations were analysed by this procedure. The possibility of inducing mutations in cells cultured *in vitro* was independently demonstrated in three laboratories (Chu and Malling, 1968a, b; Kao and Puck, 1968a, b; Shapiro *et al.*, 1968). This kind of test is becoming increasingly favoured (Fig. 5). Treated cultured cells are plated, and in general manipulated as micro-organisms. Several methods aim to investigate the so-called 'point' mutations, i.e. those that do not deal with chromosome damage, directly visible under the microscope. These latter tests will be discussed in the next chapter (group III). Modifications of the techniques according to the chemical nature of the mutagen, as well as experimental conditions have been described on several occasions for Chinese hamster (see Krooth *et al.*, 1968; Chu in Vogel and Röhrborn, 1970; Chu, 1971b). These procedures are based on the use of genetic markers which can be revealed at the cellular level. Use was made of morphological characters as well as biochemical (including nutritional mutants as in lower organisms) and serological properties and resistance to drugs or radiation.

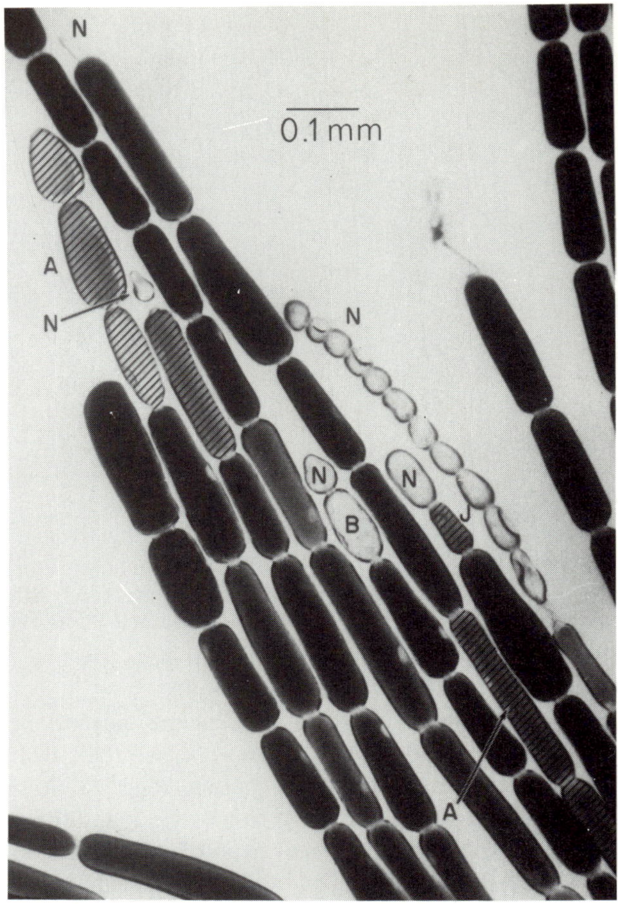

Fig. 4. Staminal hairs of *Tradescantia paludosa* showing anthocyanic mutant cells (A hatched) and abnormal cells (N) obtained after irradiation. (Picture by courtesy of Dr. A. Sparrow, Brookhaven National Laboratory, with the permission of Plenum Press.)

A special class of mutants called 'conditional lethal' makes use of cells that can form colonies in specific conditions only, but die in other conditions. Limiting factors are numerous such as nutritional components, various physical conditions such as pH, temperature, osmotic pressure, etc. In principle, all types of mammalian cells including human cells could be tested, but only after stabilization of the cell lines. One can even take advantage of tissues from organisms suffering from hereditary diseases. Such is the case of tissues of patients suffering from xeroderma pigmentosum, who show extreme sensitivity to ultraviolet (UV) irradiation which acts in this test system as a selective agent (Cleaver, 1968, 1969; Setlow *et al.*, 1969).

Attempts were made to validate gene-locus mutation assays in diploid human lymphoblast lines (Thilly *et al.*, 1980). These cell lines can easily be obtained from existing repositories and stabilized. In this test, the colony-forming ability of human lymphoblasts is determined on special feeder layers of

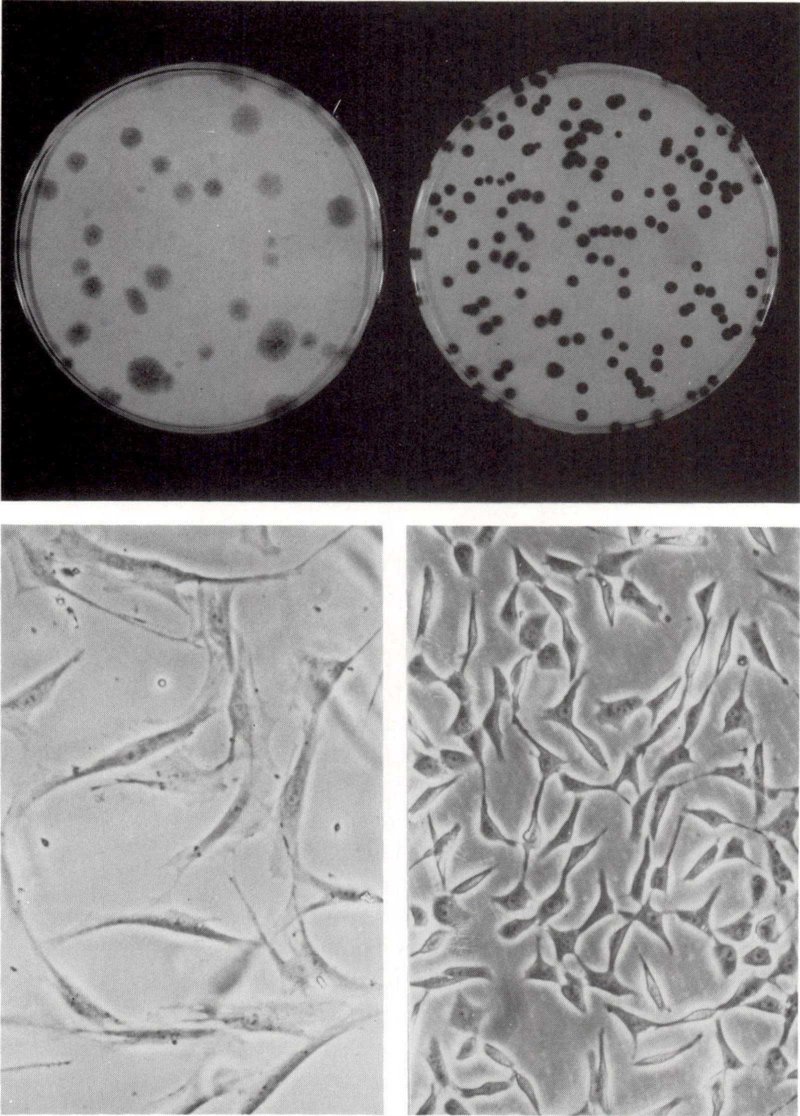

FIG. 5. *Above*. Petri dishes showing colonies of cultured mammalian cells. Left: normal human fibroblasts. Right: lung cells of Chinese hamster (line V79). *Below*. Left: human fibroblasts observed by phase contrast microscopy (× 400). Right: Chinese hamster cells (line V79) observed by phase contrast microscopy (× 400). (Pictures by courtesy of Dr. E. Chu, Department of Human Genetics, Medical School, The University of Michigan, Ann Arbor.)

fibroblasts under selective conditions, e.g. to detect 6-thioguanine-resistant or other biochemical mutants.

In recent years, immunological techniques have been used to detect cells of rare genotypes. It will be seen in Chapter 2 that there are many good methods to detect mutations at the chromosome level either *in vivo* or *in vitro*. In contrast, there are few systems available to detect gene mutations of single cells. In fact, the only tissues for experimental work in mammels or designed for monitoring human populations are blood and sperm. Immunological methods are based on the fact that mutated proteins can acquire modified antigenic properties. It is therefore possible to induce experimentally an antibody for the mutant antigen. If this antibody reacts only with the mutant protein, i.e. the mutated antigen, it is possible to measure the small proportion of mutated protein in the large amount of normal proteins. The number of mutational events can be calculated from these data.

The first requirement of these tests is to obtain monospecific antibodies in the serum by several rather elaborate techniques. A new approach is based on the possibility of synthesizing monoclonal antibodies in tissue culture. This is the so-called hybridoma technique. (For a detailed review of the techniques see Melchers *et al.*, 1978.)

In the general procedure, spleen cells from immunized mice are fused (hybridized) with plasmacytoma cells by a suitable technique. Plasmacytoma cells being malignant retain the property of continuously growing for a long time, but do not synthesize antibodies arising from a non-immunized animal.

In contrast, spleen cells synthesize antibodies since they are extracted from an immunized animal, but are unable to grow continuously not being malignant. The hybridoma which results from the fusion of the two types of cells combines both interesting properties. However, very few clones of cells will produce the specific antibody. Therefore, these clones should be properly selected and then isolated for mass production of the desired antibody.

In blood, the most widely used is the haemoglobin test system which yields interesting information on the biochemistry of this molecule. An antiserum against haemoglobin of a specific mouse strain is obtained by injecting a suitable mammal (not necessarily a mouse). Purified antibodies can be made fluorescent by coupling with a fluorochrome, generally fluorescein isothiocyanate. A blood smear of another mouse strain which does not cross-react with the haemoglobin of the strain taken as antigen is allowed to react with the fluorescent antibody. Only those red blood cells that mutated to the first strain (taken as antigen) will show fluorescence. In this test system, millions of red blood cells should be screened, a requirement which lead to the development of automated procedures to count cells. This can be performed by flow cytometry (the so-called fluorescence-activated cell sorter or FACS). Thanks to an elaborate detection system, the apparatus not only counts the cells but also separates the fluorescent mutant cells from the normal non-fluorescent cells.

The proportion of mutants can also be counted by radioimmunoassay. In this technique, red blood cells are haemolysed. Thus, abnormal molecules are counted rather than abnormal cells as in the previous technique. Radioimmunoassay is very sensitive since a proportion as small as one abnormal molecule per million normal molecules can be detected.

In sperm, several immunofluorecence test systems have been worked out. One of them concerns the detection of lactate dehydrogenase. This enzyme occurs in different forms in the spermatozoa, one of them being lactate dehydrogenase X. In mouse and also in man, the isozyme exists only in a single molecular form. This is not the case in other mammals. An antibody against rat lactate dehydrogenase is prepared by injecting a rabbit. This antibody is made fluorescent by coupling with a fluorochrome as above. Normally, the antibody should not bind with mouse sperm (rat lactate dehydrogenase not being the same as that in mouse) except for the rare mutant spermatozoa which acquired an antigenic structure similar to that of the rat. Thus, the frequency of mutants can be measured by counting the number of fluorescent spermatozoa. This test system is made more difficult by the uneven distribution of lactate dehydrogenase in and on spermatozoa. With fluorescence microscopy, non-mutant spermatozoa appear unstained. The frequency of fluorescent mutant spermatozoa is of the order of 0.43 per million with large variations depending on the strain (Ansari and Malling, 1982).

Other related test systems have also been worked out, but have not been much developed so far for technical reasons. The major histocompatibility locus (H_2) of mouse has been recommended either by using tissue-graft rejection (survey in Klein, 1978, and Bailey, 1979) or by using specific antibodies against H_2 alloantigens. The spontaneous frequency of such mutations ranges from 0.256 to 1.08 per 100 mice (Kohn and Melvold, 1974). If these immunological methods can be made a little more routine they will probably be of help in the future.

At present, attempts are being made to work out other specific immunological tests using a lectin from plants — concanavalin A. This lectin has sperm-agglutinating properties. The method is based on the detection of mutant spermatozoa that have lost surface molecules and thus their agglutinating capability (Moutschen and Colizzi, unpublished data).

There are also tests designed to detect morphological sperm abnormalities, sometimes called spermatest (Hofnung and Weil, 1980). Male mammals, generally rodents, are treated by the potential mutagen then allowed to achieve a complete spermatogenic cycle. The duration of this cycle varies from one rodent to another. For unknown reasons, sperm anomalies are induced in late spermatogonia or early spermatocytes. Mice or rats should be sacrificed at the appropriate time and the sperm harvested from the ductus deferens; in other mammals such as rabbit, sperm can be collected without killing the animal.

After appropriate staining, morphological anomalies of all parts of the spermatozoa (head, middle and end pieces) are observed. Classification of the anomalies needs to be standardized for each animal species to enable comparison of data obtained from different laboratories.

The protocol should also be standardized for all parameters; e.g. age of animal, strain, spontaneous occurrence of anomalies. This test could possibly also be routinely performed in man for the analysis of occupational hazards and epidemiological studies (Chapter 9). All details of such tests have been reviewed (Wyrobek and Bruce, 1978; Hofnung and Weil, 1980; Topham, 1983).

The tests described hitherto in eukaryotic cell test systems deal with point mutations. However, there are still other genetic changes which, in the past, were too often neglected for the evaluation of genetic risks. One of these risks is that of aneuploidy, which is widely observed in both lower and higher organisms. An aneuploid organism (or cell) has one or a few chromosomes more or less than the normal chromosome number of the species. These changes are of great importance. It is known that terrible human diseases such as heredodegeneracies have such an origin. There are two ways for detecting aneuploid mutants. The first is obviously to count the chromosomes. This is only possible in higher animal or plant cells where they are much larger than in lower organisms (Chapter 2). The second way is based on genetic properties that do not require chromosome counts but only the observation of phenotypic changes. In this context, test systems have been designed in eukaryotic micro-organisms to evaluate meiotic (e.g. in *Neurospora crassa, Sordaria brevicollis* and *Saccharomyces cerevisiae*) or mitotic (e.g. in *Saccharomyces cerevisiae* and *Aspergillus nidulans*) aneuploidy.

The last two classes of genetic changes which might be more important that mutations themselves are concerned with two fundamental genetic phenomena, namely conversion and recombination (i.e. crossing over). Doubtless, the disturbance of such processes could lead to drastic and unpredictable modifications of populations since they are more frequent events than mutations (Chapter 9). Unfortunately, the data are so scanty that they do not yet enable evaluation of the risks of such genetic changes. As regards conversion, tests are available only in a few lower eukaryotic organisms such as *Saccharomyces cerevisiae* (Moustachi, 1980). Several substances have shown convertogenic potentialities.

Nothing is known about similar induced modifications in mammals including man or about their remote genetic consequences.

Modifications of the recombination processes can be valuably analysed in eukaryotic lower organisms such as *Neurospora crassa, Saccharomyces cerevisiae* or *Schizosaccharomyces pombe.*

A multipurpose test attempting to evaluate all 'alteragenic' risks (mutagenic, convertogenic and recombinogenic) has been suggested (Moustachi, 1980).

Recently, recombinogenic effects were demonstrated in maize between three pairs of loci belonging to three different chromosome pairs after treatment with pesticides (Shoemaker and Ihrke, 1983).

Since numerous endogenous or exogenous factors are known to modify the crossing over between two loci, it is clear that future tests should include a greater number of intermediary loci. Comparable tests in mammals would

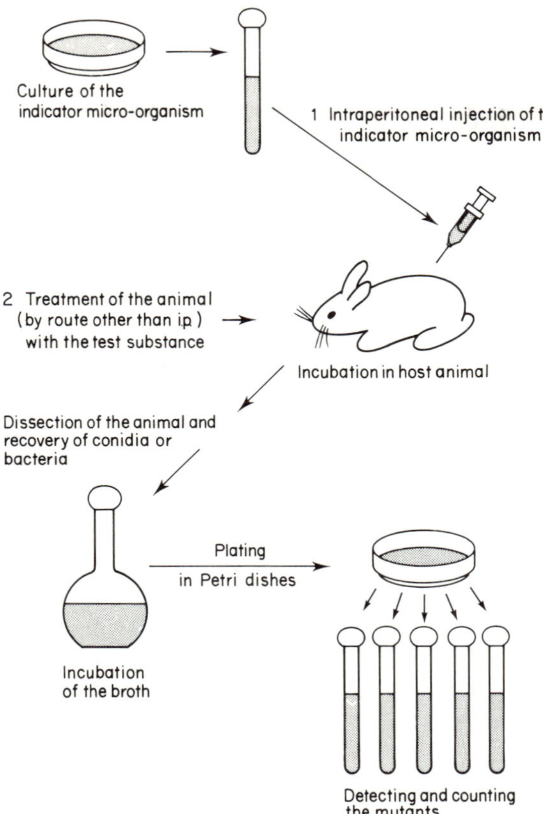

FIG. 6. Host-mediated assay procedure (according to Malling and de Serres, 1971). (Explanation in text.)

require many thousands of animals. Thus, they would be impractical if not completely unrealistic.

Indirect tests (so-called host-mediated assays) designed to investigate mutations in cell populations of lower organisms attempt to combine the advantages of lower organisms on the one hand with those of mammals on the other. They aim to detect point mutations induced not only by drugs but also by their metabolites. In fact, the mammalian organism has two parts to play in these tests: first, as the incubator, and second as the 'metabolizing system' (either activating or detoxifying).

In these tests, a broth of micro-organisms is injected into a suitably selected host (generally a mammal). The test substance is then given to the host. This substance can either be mutagenic in itself, or be activated into a real mutagen, or be detoxified by host tissues, although mutagenic in *in vitro* test systems.

After the treatment of the host, the micro-organisms are recovered, plated and then submitted to genetic analysis (Fig. 6). This test, previously developed by Gabridge and Legator (1969), Gabridge *et al.* (1969) and Legator (1970) (review in Vogel and Röhrborn, 1970) was further improved according to practical requirements. First, a strain of *Salmonella typhimurium* unable to synthesize an amino acid (lysineless), was injected into the intraperitoneal cavity of a mouse. The substance under investigation was given to the mouse by a different route to avoid preferential treatment of micro-organisms before any possibility of metabolization by the host. The recovered bacteria were then plated on a suitably selected medium without lysine in such a way that only reverse mutants could grow (Fig. 6).

Several researchers have attempted to improve this technique. The use of completely non-pathogenic micro-organisms was first recommended for obvious reasons; e.g. *Neurospora* (cited by Malling and Cosgrove in Vogel and Rörhborn, 1970; description of the technique in Malling and de Serres, 1971, in Gen. Refs.) or *Saccharomyces* (Fahrig, 1971).

Chu and Malling (1971) used hamster cells instead of micro-organisms. There are in principle no experimental objections to using human cells of stabilized lines, but there still seems to be real difficulty for many lines. Another modification of the host-mediated assay is to inject cells to be treated in a specific place in the host, e.g. kidney, liver or testicle. In this way, one could possibly obtain a more homogeneous and reproducible response and an easier recovery. By comparing different assays, one can also get an idea of the efficiency of the barriers that prevent the free diffusion of the substances in the organism, especially in gonads. The significance of the tests and the conditions under which they can be applied will be discussed in Chapter 3.

Chapter 2

Methodology for Detecting Clastogenic Effects and Mutations at the Level of the Entire Organism

Subdivision of the classical methodology into two chapters seems somewhat arbitrary since tests for detecting chromosome damage could as well be classified in group II (Chapter 1) which includes mutation tests at the cellular level. However, since chromosome damage does not inevitably result in a mutation (see below) and requires a particular microscopic technique different from the techniques used in tests of group II, we classify these so-called tests of clastogenicity (from the Greek χλαστος — broken and γενεσις — the (act of) generation) in a separate group (group III).

Group III

Under this heading are grouped all chromosomal aberrations that are visible microscopically. Some aberrations are actually breaks; others involve repair processes and are chromosome rearrangements. They are sometimes called, rightly or wrongly, 'radiomimetic' aberrations, because ionizing radiations first allowed their detailed investigation (description in various textbooks or papers: Kaufmann in Hollaender, 1954; Giles in Hollaender, 1954; Swanson in Swanson, 1957, in Gen. Refs.; Evans, 1962; Lewis and John, 1963, in Gen. Refs.; Kihlman, 1966, in Gen. Refs.; Rieger and Michaelis, 1967, in Gen. Refs.; Evans in Hollaender, 1976).

The complexity of the problems is sometimes such that studies of chromosome breakage form almost a true branch of genetics. In short, in all these tests, cell populations, as homogeneous as possible, are treated for a period covering a part of or a whole mitotic cycle or even several successive cycles. Then the chromosome damage is detected and estimated with the best microscopic techniques available.

Diffuse lesions such as chromosome clumping or stickiness, which are indicative of cytotoxicity not necessarily correlated with genotoxicity, can lead to cell death or recovery without alteration of the genomes. Inversely, minor chromosomal lesions which correspond to true mutations do not inevitably produce the death of the cell. There is no comprehensive treatise exclusively devoted to clastogenicity, but there are general textbooks dealing in detail with the most important problems (see above). In the past, their genetic significance, i.e. the chances of the lesions resulting in true mutations without being eliminated, was not always fully understood.

We have proposed a classification of chromosomal damage based on the following guidelines (Moutschen, 1970):

(1) Major losses of chromatin have a greater chance of being selected out during the successive mitotic cycles following the treatment or during the developmental processes of the treated organism and its progeny, because they carry a higher risk of producing the death of the cell. Therefore, if these short- or long-term cytotoxic effects occur, they have no genetic consequences. As in many pathological processes, the elimination of the lesion is in some ways a kind of defence reaction of the carrier organism. When the damage can not be repaired, it is rejected (Fig. 7).

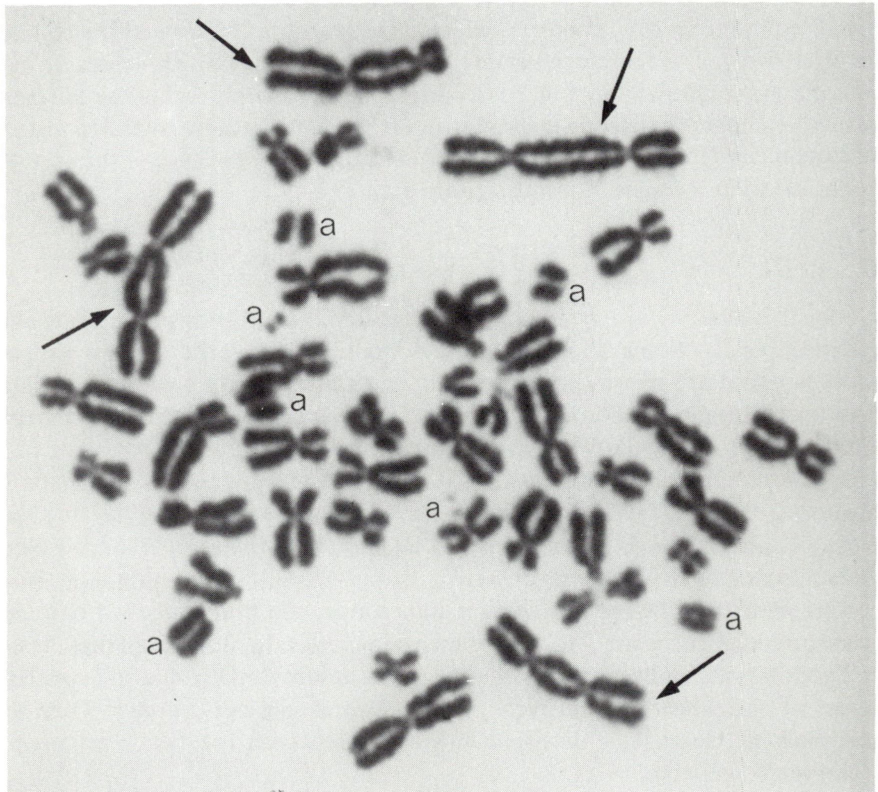

FIG. 7. Chromosome damage due to mutagenic agents.
A cultured human lymphocyte exposed to X-rays (about 300 rads) showing several chromosome aberrations. Dicentric chromosomes are indicated by arrows. These asymmetric translocations result in major losses of chromatin (a indicates acentric fragments) (× 3400)
Because of this significant radio-induced damage, this cell-line is likely to degenerate (Picture by courtesy of M.-C. Chollet, Laboratoire de Cytogénétique, Dr. A. Léonard, Centre d'Energie Nucléaire, Mol.)

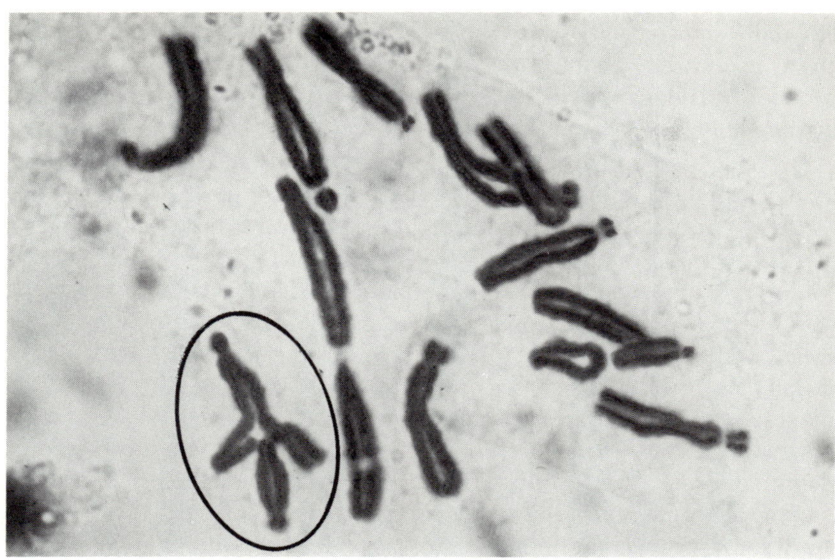

FIG. 8. Chromosome damage due to mutagenic agents.
Root-tip cell of broad bean treated with Myleran (mM, 3 h) showing various aberrations of the chromatid type. A symmetrical translocation (quadriradial) configuration) is encircled. This lesion can result in meiotic mispairing (as shown in Fig. 17) producing sterility (× 2200) (Picture: Dr. J. Moutschen.)

(2) Only symmetrical aberrations (Fig. 8) do not produce major losses of chromatin, and can result in favourable or unfavourable mutations (this is unpredictable).
(3) There are specific segments of chromosomes where lesions occur more frequently, and for which the risk of mutation is much higher. Some chemicals seem to have a specific affinity for chromosomal segments of crucial importance.

In plants, almost all types of organs could be used in test systems to estimate chromosomal damage. However, root tips, pollen grains and pollen mother-cells are generally preferred.

Plant tissue cultures suitable for solving a wide range of problems do not seem to be so valuable for investigating chromosome breakage, especially because of frequent endopolyploidy leading to high chromosome numbers, and also due to lack of homogeneity of cultured cell populations. In mammals, series of experiments have been performed *in vitro* as well as *in vivo*. A great variety of cells, the karyotypic stability of which has been previously verified, can serve this purpose; in particular can be mentioned fibroblasts (Harnden, 1960), lymphocytes (Hirschhorn, 1965), kidney cells of several primate species (Bender and Chu, 1963; Chu and Bender, 1964), bone marrow cells (Tjio and Whang, 1962), amniotic cells (Legator *et al.*, 1978) and even ascites tumour cells (for a review, see Adler, 1970). In contrast, in mouse, the best known mammal for genetic investigations, the stabilization of cell lines is still difficult

(Chu and Monesi, 1960). One essential point in all these tests is to select cells with sufficiently large chromosomes and relatively low chromosome numbers. Moreover, it is desirable though not mandatory for all purposes to be able to identify each chromosome separately. There are no objections to the use of human lines, save for difficulties of stabilization as stated in Chapter 1. As regards chromosome breakage, the rapid improvement of techniques during the last two decades has allowed some problems to be approached which had hitherto remained totally unresolved (Fig. 9).

Meiotic chromosome analysis in mammals *in vivo* has been refined and has certainly become more relevant. Two kinds of analysis can be carried out in parallel, at the diakinesis–metaphase stages at which bivalents are widespread and details of the chromosomes are quite visible (see Fig. 18). Chromosome damage can also be analysed at other meiotic stages such as spermatocytic anaphases I and II. Although the damage will be underestimated on account of the elimination of a proportion of the aberrations from metaphase to anaphase, this method would still be valuable for rapid screening.

Another improvement in the field of clastogenicity studies is the possibility of investigating chromosome damage in oocytes. This is based on the well-known use of hormones to induce ovulation at the time desired (Jagiello, 1965) and then to inject colchicine, thus allowing examination of metaphase I instead of the more difficult metaphase II (Tarkowski, 1966).

Despite these technical improvements, there are still relatively few studies which describe damage induced in females, and the treatments were generally performed with strong mutagens such as X-rays (Caine and Lyon, 1977) or alkylating agents (Brewen and Payne, 1976, 1978).

In parallel with classical tests of clastogenicity, three tests have been recommended and are now becoming increasingly used either as additional tests or for routine screening of a lot of chemicals. The first test — the micronucleus test — analyses the damage resulting from previously induced chromosome breakage. The second is based on the examination of sister-chromatid exchanges. The third, more recent, test groups together some tests designed to investigate chromosome non-disjunction at the microscopic level.

The micronucleus test (Fig. 10) was developed by Schmid and coworkers (review in Schmid, 1976; Jenssen and Ramel, 1980), and is based on the following principles: when a chromosome is broken, if the acentric fragment is not reincorporated into a daughter nucleus, it lags between the poles and is generally transformed into a nucleus, smaller than the main nucleus and called a micronucleus. Micronuclei have been described in classical haematology under the name Howell-Jolly bodies.

After treatment with chemical mutagens, such micronuclei can be observed in several mammal bone marrow cell lines as myeloblasts, myelocytes, erythroblasts and erythrocytes provided that the cytoplasm is sufficiently contrasted. Young erythrocytes are generally selected for counting micronuclei, which remain in the cell after the main nuclei are expelled.

Sister-chromatid exchanges (Fig. 11) were first observed by Taylor (1958)

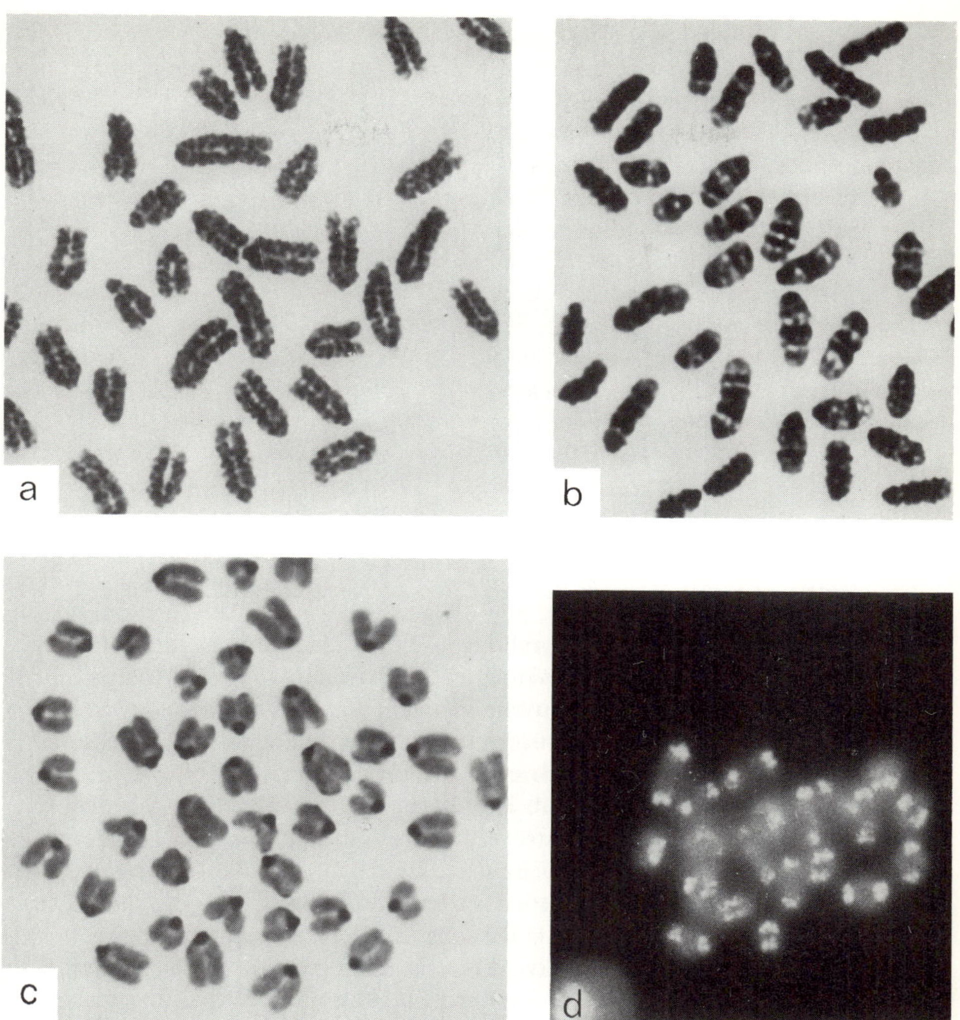

FIG. 9. Some methods of analysing chromosome damage.
a. Induced chromosome despiralization in a bone marrow cell of mouse by immersion in a hypotonic solution (containing potassium chloride and potassium acetate) then stained by Feulgen. This technique facilitates the detection of some lesions (× 1600).
b. Induction of G banding (G for Giemsa) in a spermatogonium of mouse by immersion in a hypotonic solution (containing sodium chloride and sodium acetate) then stained with Giemsa. This technique improves the localization of some chromosome aberrations (× 1600).
c. Induction of C (centromeric) banding in a bone marrow cell of mouse obtained by thermal denaturation followed by Giemsa staining. Centromeric regions are more deeply stained which allows the detection of lesions localized in these areas (× 1500).
d. Induction of bands localized at the terminal regions of chromosome bivalents during mouse spermatogenesis. These bands are obtained after differential enzymatic digestion followed by acridine orange staining. Observations by fluorescence microscopy (Pictures: Dr. J. Moutschen.) (× 1250)

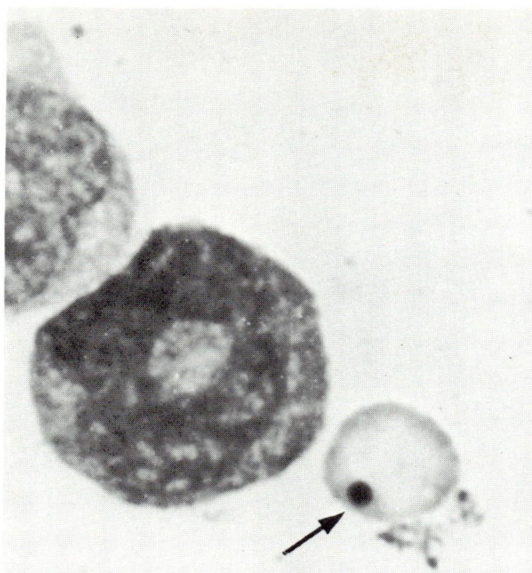

FIG. 10. Example of micronucleus (arrowed) in a mouse erythroblast. (Picture by courtesy of Dr. A. Léonard, Centre d'Energie Nucléaire, Mol.) (× 2000)

after incorporation of tritiated thymidine into the chromosomes. Most of them were probably induced by the radioactivity of tritium. It was further established that by incorporating a pyrimidine analogue, 5-bromodeoxyuridine (BUdR), into the chromosome, sister-chromatid exchange formation requires at least one replication cycle. Briefly, the procedure is as follows in cells cultured *in vitro,* e.g. mammalian lymphocytes. After exposure for a short period to the test agent, cells are treated with BUdR for one replication cycle and illuminated. The interaction of light and BUdR induce SCE. After harvesting and fixation, they are stained either by a fluorescent dye (e.g. Hoechst 33250). It was observed that BUdR substituted chromatids fluoresce less efficiently than normal chromatids. This permits detection of the exchange points. Staining chromatids with Giemsa is now used more than fluorescent stains in routine tests. The procedure has been adapted to test systems *in vivo*, e.g. mouse (Allen and Latt, 1976; Vogel and Bauknecht, 1976) or chick (Bloom and Hsu, 1975). (For a review of technical details on sister-chromatid exchanges see Latt and Allen, 1977.)

Group II (Chapter 1) includes a series of tests designed to reveal aneuploidy in mutant phenotypes. Group III includes some tests aimed at detecting aneuploidy but on the basis of microscopic observations. Mitotic or meiotic aneuploidy is certainly easy to observe in higher plants, but since these test systems generally show a high frequency of partial (aneuploidy) or total polyploidy, the interpretation of the data collected in plants is somewhat difficult. This is possibly a reason why meiotic analysis of aneuploidy was carried out in various mammals. The frequency of such anomalies was found to fluctuate somewhat from species to species. In rodents, Hansmann and Probeck (1979) reported a frequency of aneuploid zygotes of less than 1%, which is said to be a low spontaneous level though fairly high compared with other mutations.

FIG. 11. Technique for showing sister-chromatid exchanges in human cultured lymphocytes. After incorporation of bromodeoxyuridine (10 µg/ml) for one mitotic cycle, chromatids are stained with Giemsa.
a. Untreated (control) lymphocyte to show the background. One chromatid is more stained by few sister-chromatid exchanges are visible (indicated by the arrow).

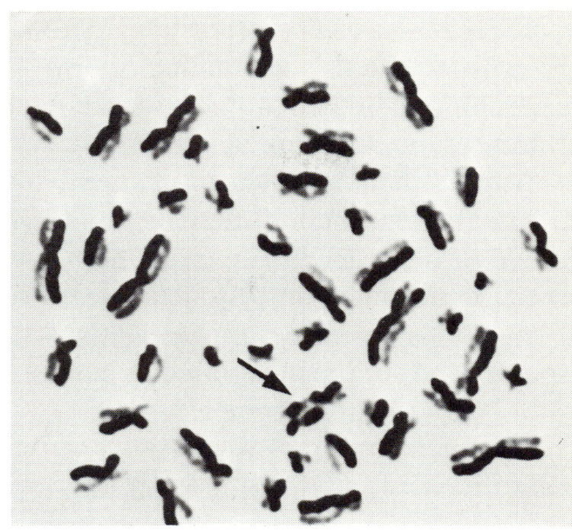

a

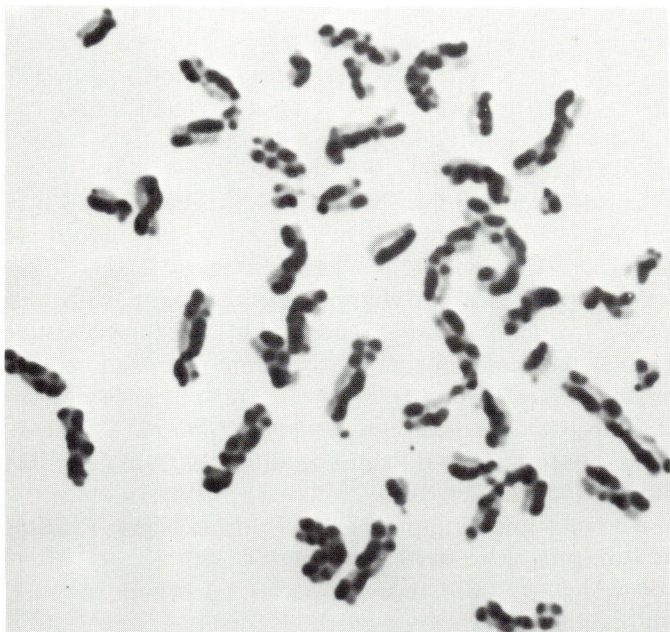

b

b. Cell treated with cyclophosphamide 1×10^{-4} M. (a promutagen after activation by microsomal fraction into a true mutagen). The number of sister-chromatid exchanges is extremely enhanced. Chromosomes are named *harlequin*. (× 3400). (Pictures due to the courtesy of Dr. A. Léonard, Centre d'Energie Nucléaire, Mol)

In man, a large proportion of early abortions are known to be aneuploid. This observation stimulated interesting investigations of this class of anomalies in another primate, the marmoset (*Callithix jacchus*). A frequency of aneuploid zygotes as high as 4% was reported (Bobrow and Ejiwunmi, 1978). The interpretation of these data is obscured by particularities of the fertilization, leading to an overestimation of the frequency and making comparison with human data difficult.

There is also a very interesting approach for monitoring human populations. It consists simply of staining sperm with a fluorescent probe, and then examining them with a fluorescence microscope. In normal sperm, the Y sex chromosome is visible as a fluorescent body (F body) always located at the same place behind the head of spermatozoon (Beatty, 1977). The occurrence of two fluorescent bodies in the same head is interpreted as non-disjunction of the Y chromosomes. The frequency of such an anomaly is a biased measure of the chromosome non-disjunction occurring in the human population. Animal populations can also be investigated with this technique. Unfortunately, the sperm heads of the most familiar animal for genetic studies — mouse — do not show fluorescent Y bodies.

Chromosomal non-disjunctions can also be analysed in whole-body tests (e.g. in *Drosophila* and mouse) for sex chromosomes (see below).

Group IV

This group includes a wide variety of tests performed on the most diverse organisms. The genetic system peculiar to each organism or group of organisms should first be taken into account. In plants, seeds are the organs treated in the majority of cases. Following the pioneering observations of Stadler (1928) in maize and of Gustafsson (1940, 1947, in Gen. Refs.) in barley, research by the Swedish school of mutagenesis (Nilan, 1964, in Gen. Refs.; Ehrenberg, 1971; Nilan and Vig, 1976) aimed first at estimating the induced sterility at the treated generation (M_1) and at the subsequent one (M_2) (Fig. 12). At this latter generation, morphological and chlorophyll mutants (i.e. with damage to genes governing the synthetic pathways required for chloroplast development) were investigated at the same time as the spectrum of mutations. This and some related methods have been extended to other plant species such as maize, broad bean, pea and *Arabidopsis thaliana* (National Academy of Science 'Symposium on Mutation and Plant Breeding', 1961, in Gen. Refs.; Hagberg and Åkerberg, 1962, in Gen. Refs.; Röbbelen, 1964). In wheat (hexaploids for *Triticum aestivum* and tetraploids for *T. durum* and *T. dicoccum*), very powerful mutagens were particularly tested, due to the buffering effect of polyploidy (MacKey, 1967). In some species, floral buds were treated and the effects on the progeny were recorded.

In an attempt to increase the resolving power of the tests and at the same time make them easier to perform, somatic mutations of various plants were proposed as test systems. It is known that when a cell mutates at an early stage of development (e.g. the plant embryo within the seed), this mutant cell gives rise to a lineage of mutant cells that eventually result in a whole mutant sector visible either with the naked eye or a lens. In this context, an elegant test was worked out in maize (Fig. 13). The principle of the test is as follows: a stock of plants heterozygous for the *yg2 (yellow-green 2)* gene is first developed. The leaves have a normal colour, the recessive *yg2* gene being completely masked by its normal allele. When kernels are treated by mutagenic agents at concentrations suitably chosen to allow normal germination, the wild allele of the *yg2* gene can be 'inactivated' with a certain frequency. In this case, the gene *yg2* can

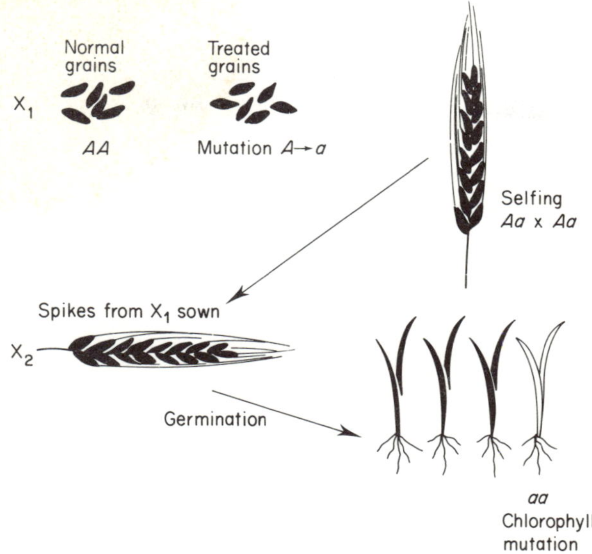

FIG. 12. Method designed to detect chlorophyll mutations in barley (according to Gustafsson). Barley caryopses of the treated generation (X_1) are sown. Induced sterility is investigated in spikes arising from these caryopses. Spikes of X_1 are sown, and at the generation X_2 chlorophyll mutations are scored. This test can be extended to other cereals. Morphological mutations, recessive and viable, can also be recorded at a third generation

appear, giving rise to a cell streak of a yellow-green colour, easily seen through a lens against the green background of the leaves. The frequency of each mutagenic event can then be estimated with some precision.

These test systems can in some ways be compared to those which aim to detect mutations in pollen or staminal hairs (group I; see Chapter 1).

Among the multiplicity of tests now available in group IV, a special place should be ascribed to the tests developed during the last decades in animals. In *Drosophila,* all kinds of mutations have been extensively worked out. The possibility of obtaining large stocks at relatively low cost explains why *Drosophila* has been so popular. General tests (for each kind of mutation) and tests designed to investigate chromosomal rearrangements can be distinguished.

The first group comprises sex-linked mutations (recessive, lethal and visible). Among the most routinely used, we can mention *ClB*, *Muller-5* (Fig. 14), *B In sc y* and attached *X*. There are also tests for autosomic recessive, lethal and visible mutations. Some tests were even intended to estimate cumulative effects for successive generations (e.g. *facl*/female accumulation of lethal mutations). Others, like the multipurpose test, attempt to detect various types of mutations simultaneously. All of these tests are based on the use of so-called 'synthetic' chromosomes especially constructed for the purpose of mutation studies. The morphological characteristics selected are suitable and easy to observe. All details of these tests and of others more elaborate have been amply described (Muller and Oster in Burdette, 1963). An efficient test to

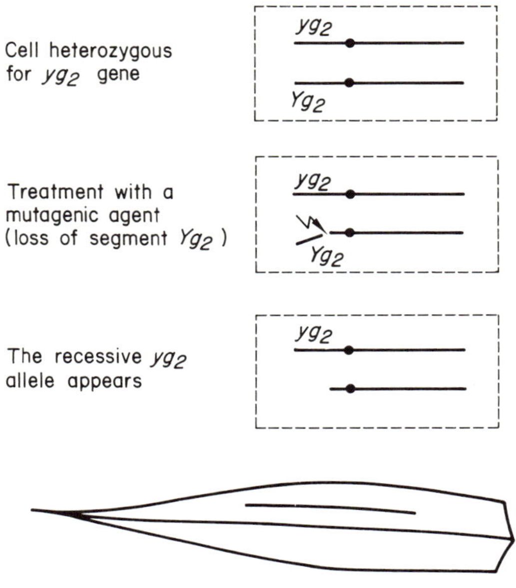

FIG. 13. *yg2* test in maize (explanation in the text).

detect dominant lethal mutations, considered to be of chromosomal origin was worked out by Telfer (1954). Some genetic techniques allow the frequency of chromosome aberrations in *Drosophila* to be determined, including loss and gains of chromosomes, particularly sex chromosomes (Brosseau *et al.*, 1961; Lindsley and Grell, 1967).

Other insects (e.g. *Habrobracon juglandis* and *Ephestia kühniella*) are also available for mutagenicity testing although the techniques are generally not so elaborate as in *Drosophila* (review of *E. kühniella* in Whiting, 1961; review of the techniques for the two other organisms in Smith and von Borstel, 1971).

Mutagenicity tests on whole mammals have been preferentially performed on mice. As in *Drosophila,* we can distinguish between general tests and others more specifically designed to investigate chromosomal aberrations.

The seven-locus test worked out by Russel (1951) is based on the following principles (review in Cattanach, 1971; Ehling, 1978). A stock of mice, homozygous for the specific genes is developed: *a (non-agouti), b (brown),* c^{ch} *(chinchilla), d (dilute), se (short ear), p (pink eyed dilution), s (piebald spotting)*. Being recessive and normally masked by the wild dominant alleles, these genes do not appear at the first generation after mating wild type with the strain homozygous for the seven loci. When a mutation of the wild gene is induced, the character appears at the first generation, allowing the detection of the mutation (Fig. 15). In practice, wild type males are treated by the mutagen under investigation, then mated with females homozygous for the seven loci. Mutations are recovered at the first generation. Since mutations are rare events, and since a small number of genes are tested, tens and even hundreds of

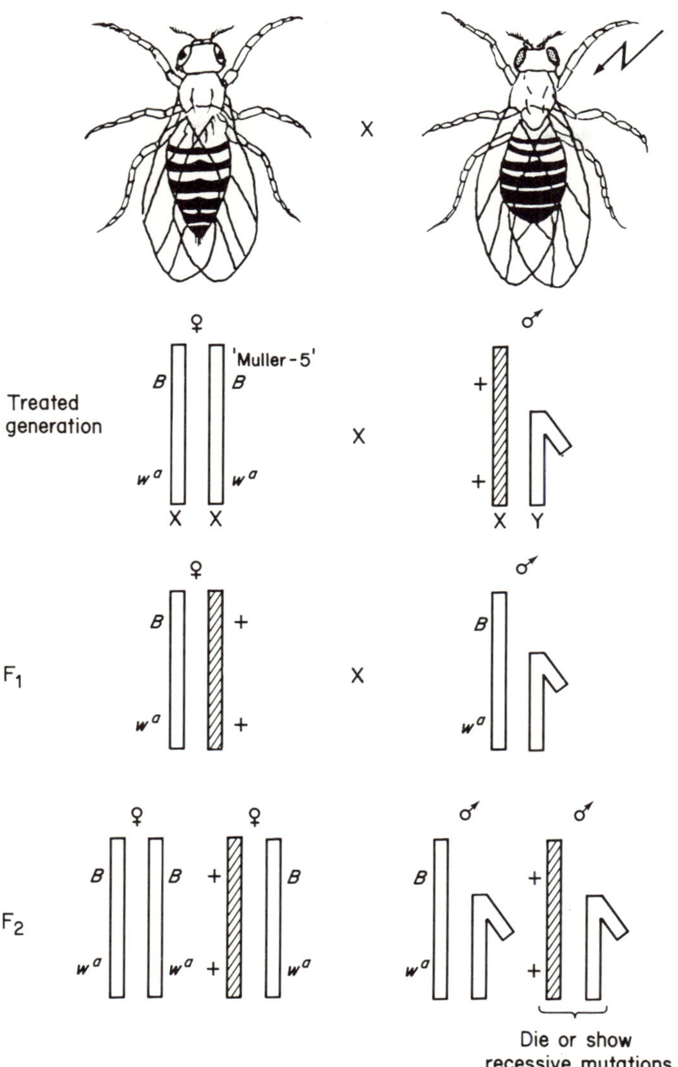

FIG. 14. Muller-5 test in *Drosophila*.
Males (♂) with an X sex chromosome tested (hatched) are treated with the agent investigated, then mated with females (♀) with the chromosome Muller-5. This X chromosome has a specific chromosome rearrangement and two sex-linked genes, respectively *B* (*Bar*), an eye mutation, and w^a (*white apricot*), another eye mutation. Dominant mutation can be detected at the first generation (F_1). F_1 flies mated individually *inter se* give four classes in F_2. F_2 males with the treated X chromosomes die if a recessive lethal gene has been induced or reveal recessive visible mutations since these linked genes have no counterpart in the Y chromosome. Results can be confirmed with an F_3

thousands of mice are necessary to obtain reliable results. This test has been applied to chemical mutagens (Ehling, 1970, 1978; Russel *et al.*, 1981a).

This method was somewhat modified by Lyon and Morris (1966, 1969) using

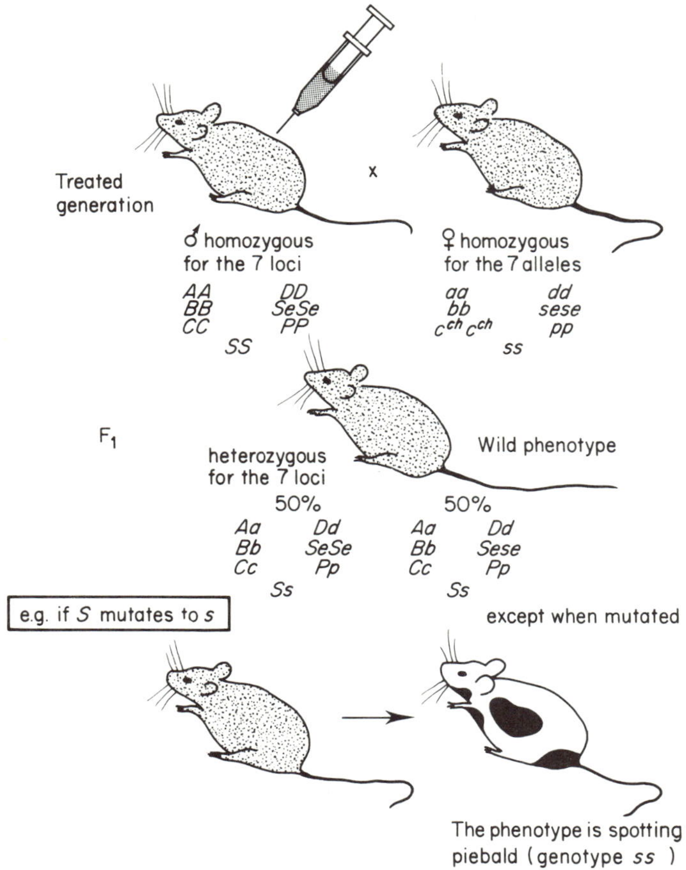

FIG. 15. Mouse seven-locus test (explanation in the text)

a stock of mice containing genes *a (non-agouti)*, *bp (brachypodism)*, *fz (fuzzy)*, *ln (leaden)*, *pa (pallid)*, and *pe (pearl)* selected on the basis of their spontaneous mutability being lower than in the Russel test.

The spot test is another *in vivo* method for detecting somatic mutations in mice. In principle, it could be extended to other mammals. It is based on the pioneer experiment of Russel and Major (1957) who observed induced colour mosaics in mouse embryos after X-irradiation of specific strains.

In 1974–1975, stocks especially devised for this test were multiplied in several laboratories. The procedure is as follows: males of an *a/a (non-agouti)* stock but otherwise wild are mated with mice of the so-called T stock which contains the recessive genes used in the seven-locus test, so that the embryos are heterozygous for such genes and therefore do not show the recessive coat colour genes. These embryos are treated *in utero* between day 7 and day 10 of pregnancy, generally by intraperitoneal injection into the mother. If a precursor cell of the wild type gene mutates, then the recessive gene can express itself in the progeny (14-day-old young) as a spot of various colours and sizes. This is, in fact, the same general method as described for the seven-locus test (for details see Fahrig, 1978; Russel *et al.*, 1981b).

The mammalian spot test is in one respect comparable to the yellow-green (*yg2*) test in maize, being a test which detects somatic mutations. It is mentioned here because it is derived from the seven-locus test.

Biochemical specific-locus mutations can also be induced in mammals instead of morphological mutations. The main biochemical markers used by now are glucose-6-phosphate dehydrogenase, isocitrate dehydrogenase and malate dehydrogenase, some esterases, glucose phosphate isomerase, phosphoglucomutase, diaminopeptidase and haemoglobin. This study has been made possible by advances in electrophoretic and enzymatic techniques. Protein variants obtained by electrophoretic separation of complex mixtures of proteins have been demonstrated after treatments of mice with methylnitrosourea, a very strong mutagen (Klose, 1977).

It has been shown that the mutation rate of biochemical loci varies from stock to stock. For four loci (two distinct haemoglobin loci, and malate and isocitrate dehydrogenase), the mutation rate per locus per gamete induced by irradiation with ^{60}Co gamma rays (2 × 500 R at 24 h intervals) in DBA mouse spermatogonia mated with C57BL females was 17.1×10^{-5} (Malling and Valcovic, 1977), whereas comparable irradiation of an Oak Ridge stock yielded 49.9×10^{-5} per R per locus (Russel, 1965) and of a Harwell stock 13.5×10^{-5} only (Lyon and Morris, 1969). For haemoglobin loci, a system was worked out combining these loci with five visible specific loci. Data are still somewhat preliminary, but suggest that for these loci the mutation rate is of the same order of magnitude as for visible loci (Russel *et al.*, 1976).

The use of biochemical specific loci is certainly of great interest not only to elucidate various problems of environmental mutagenesis, but also to investigate the nature of mutations induced by several agents, since molecular details of the gene products can be rather easily identified. The use of the biochemical specific-locus mutation system can also be extended to epidemiological studies in man (Chapter 9).

Quite different tests have also been recommended in mouse. They are in some ways comparable to the tests performed in *Drosophila* for chromosome non-disjunction of sex chromosomes. They make use of sex-linked 'markers' such as the *Tabby* gene (Russel and Saylors, 1963; Moutschen, 1969), and also the fact that the female mouse which has only one X chromosome (the so-called XO female) is morphologically normal and fertile. This is not the case in the corresponding Turner syndrome in man (for a review, see Russel in Hollaender, 1976).

The dominant lethality test was first successfully used to measure mutagenic effects of ionizing radiations by Russel *et al.* (1954) and then by Bateman (1958a, b). It has since been extended to other mammals such as rat and hamster. Initially, treated animals (one sex or other or both sexes) are mated. The time of fertilization is pin-pointed by an appropriate technique depending on the animal species. Females are then sacrificed in the second part of the

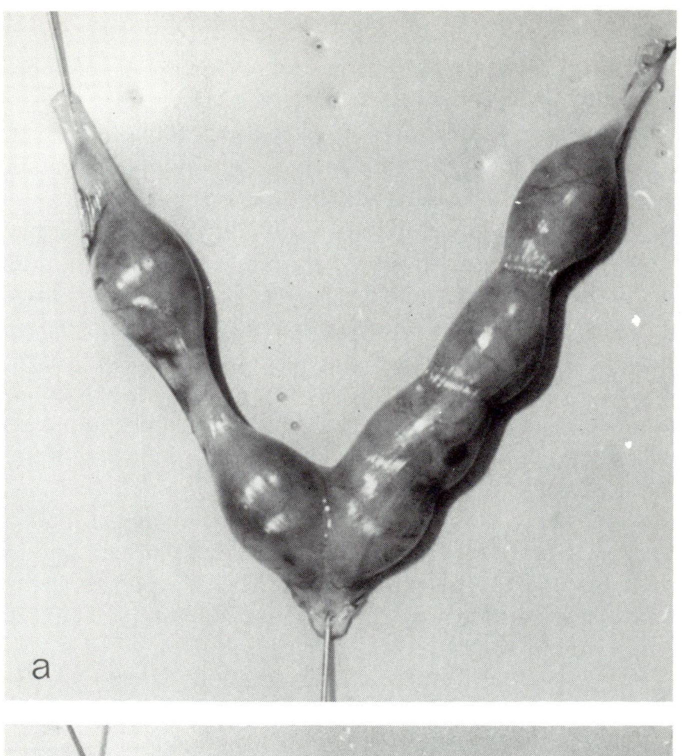

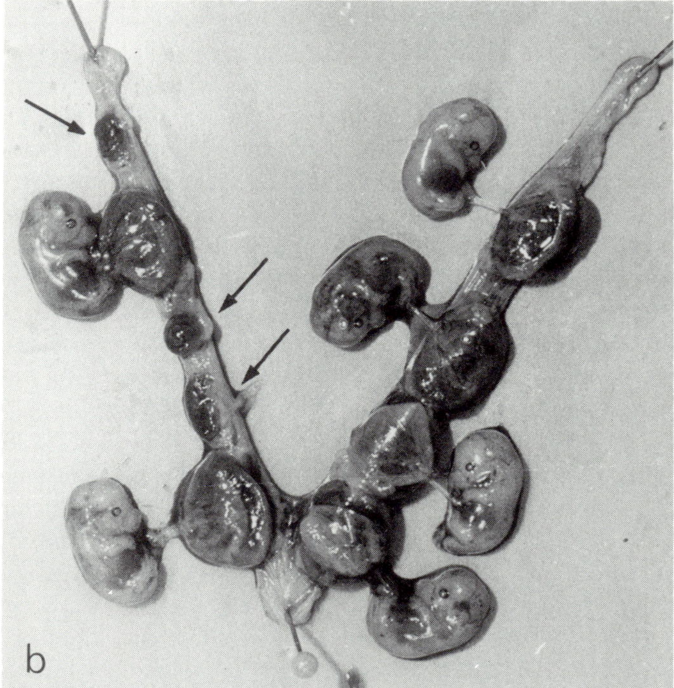

FIG. 16. Dominant lethal mutation test in mouse (explanation in the text).
a. Uterus at day 15 of pregnancy.
b. Uterus after dissection: six live young are visible; deciduomata which represent post-implantation lethal mutations are indicated by arrows

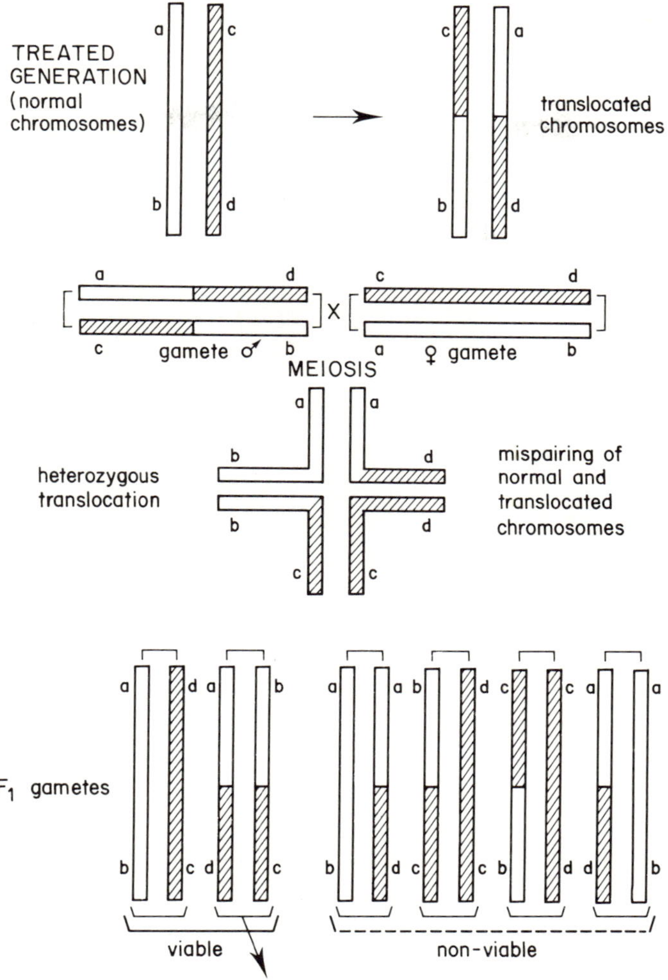

FIG. 17. Test of heritable translocation (explanation in the text)

gestation period, always at the same time, suitably selected (Fig. 16). The number of live young are counted as well as the corpora lutea of pregnancy which, in general, correspond to the number of fertilized ovulae. Then the number of degenerating embryos (deciduomata) is counted; this evaluates post-implantation death. The record can be completed by evaluating pre-implantation losses, deducting from the number of corpora lutea the sum of the young alive plus the post-implantation deaths. Methods have been worked out to calculate correctly the frequency of dominant lethal mutations and to make an appropriate statistical estimation (Röhrborn, 1970; Krüger, 1970).

Among the genetic tests designed to measure the frequency of chromosomal rearrangements, the test of heritable translocation is almost the only one practically performed (Fig. 17) on a sufficiently large scale to be relevant. It is

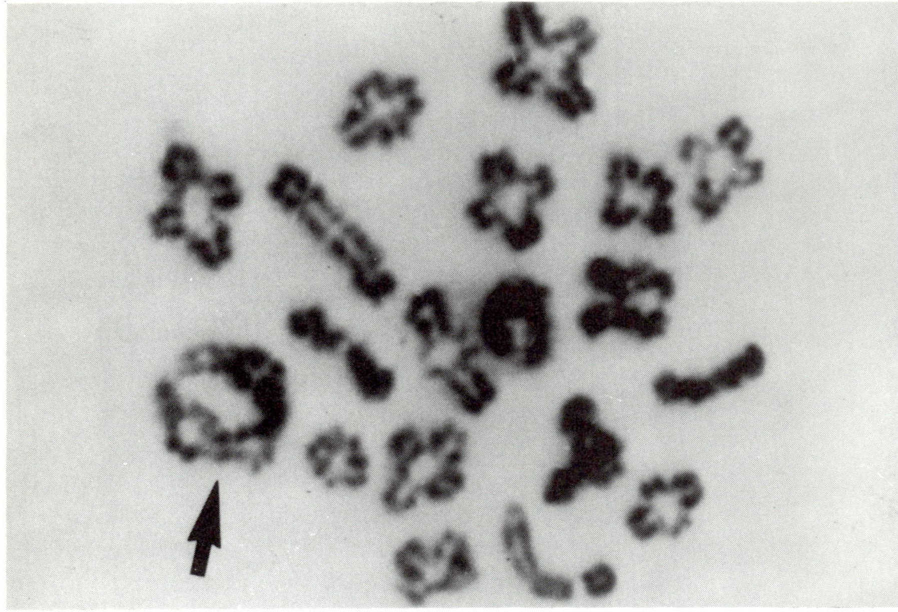

FIG. 18. Chromosome translocation observed in mouse spermatogenesis. Eighteen normally paired bivalent chromosome are counted. Abnormal pairing by four (arrowed) allows the translocation to be detected. The male carrier of this lesion had been irradiated with ionizing radiation. (Picture by courtesy of Dr. A. Malashenko, Laboratory of Experimental Biological Models, Moscow.) (× 2600)

based on the fact that animals carrying a heterozygous chromosomal translocation (see also group II) are poorly or not at all fertile. Half of the progeny (hemisterility) should theoretically contain the translocation and in turn show reduced fertility. This is not often the case, however, and large variations of fertility are commonly observed. In practice, animals of the treated generation are mated to untreated females. Their progeny, carefully collected, are tested; each animal of this generation is individually crossed with a partner from a controlled stock, free of spontaneous chromosomal rearrangements. The progeny of the second generation is checked and each animal of the preceding generation suspected of carrying a translocation reducing the litter size (lower fertility) is submitted to cytological verification. This is best performed during spermatogenesis at diakineses or metaphases I, where pairing anomalies characterizing the translocation can be clearly observed (Fig. 18). Animals of the next generation can also be utilized for cytological controls. This test, which has the advantage of allowing a comparison between genetic and cytological data, is somewhat time-consuming, requiring two generations at least, and requires large numbers of animals and experienced investigators.

After having briefly described the methods now available for identifying mutagenic agents in the environment, we will now evaluate the significance of these tests.

Chapter 3

Towards A New Methodology

'On n'agirait pas si l'on ne se propesait un but, et l'on ne recherche une chose que parce qu'on en ressent la privation'

Henri Bergson
L'Evolution créatrice, L'Existence et le Néant

QUALITIES REQUIRED FOR TESTS OF MUTAGENICITY

(1) In the context of genetic toxicology, one of the prime qualities of the chosen method is to provide results *applicable to man,* whether or not allowing direct extrapolation from animals. In the latter case, the data arising from experiments should at any rate provide precise information about the risks for man in specified circumstances in such a way that recommendations can be made from this information. It should be pointed out that the usefulness of some tests does not go much beyond the biological material investigated. Sometimes results vary markedly from strain to strain. Because of the more direct applicability of the results to man, mammals have often been recommended as an experimental material. However, even on the basis of data collected in, for example, mouse, extrapolation of the results to man is far from being automatic. Protective and detoxifying mechanisms can interact in one mammal and not in another. These differences are of great significance in the generalization of results.

(2) Tests should be sufficiently *sensitive* to detect low quantities of mutagen in the environment. It should be remembered that the methodology utilized until now was intended to investigate the effects of extremely powerful mutagens such as ionizing radiations or alkylating agents. The aim was to obtain the highest possible effects with a mutagen, whereas the present problem is to detect potential genetic effects of various contaminants not usually present in the environment at high concentrations. Therefore, the limit of the sensitivity of the available methods is rapidly reached. The only means of coping with this difficulty is to increase, sometimes considerably, the sample size. In higher organisms, this requirement has obvious disadvantages.

Like all the tests in classical toxicology, all genetic tests must include at least one control to ascertain the level of spontaneous mutational events.

When the test substance is weakly soluble in water or saline, it is necessary to use an appropriate solvent. Therefore, a control with this solvent should be added to the test. An additional positive control has also been proposed. A parallel experiment should be carried out with an agent known to produce genetic effects in the selected test system. Selection of the substance to test as positive control is important. Whenever possible the choice should be guided by similarity of the molecular structure. A dose–response curve should also be demonstrated, ideally within the range of doses where linearity is found.

(3) The high sensitivity of the tests demands rigorous experimental planning as well as *a priori* and *a posteriori statistical analyses*, the efficiency of which must be previously tested. Mathematical models have variable implications in genetic toxicology. *A priori* statistics are first required to determine sample size as a function of the dose selected and of the background (control) level. Before beginning genetic experiments, a classical toxicological parameter should be defined. This would be the LD_{50} for higher organisms, and possibly the LD_{37} for lower organisms. The reason for this preliminary test is that determination of the maximum mutation frequency strongly depends on the toxicity level. *A priori* statistics will also help evaluate the sample size of the positive control. At this stage of the research, the mathematical models may be either stochastic, based on the assumption of a Poisson distribution of mutational events, or deterministic, based on data from the literature.

A posteriori statistics should lead eventually to assessment of the risks for man of the test substance. A quantitative evaluation can only be made by establishing the dose–response relationship. This sometimes requires a large number of 'significant' points and, as stated above, an exact knowledge of the relationship between mutation and killing (Haynes and Eckardt, 1980).

The kinetics of mutation induction should also take into account the existence of damage repair processes.

The statistical inference of genetic toxicity tests has been reviewed comparatively in various organisms: the micronucleus test in *Drosophila,* in *Salmonella typhimurium,* and in mammals; and dominant lethal mutations (Ehrenberg, 1977). The statistical efficiency varies from one test system to another. For instance, in the sex-linked lethal mutation test in *Drosophila,* the tables of Kastenbaum and Bowman (1970) are generally recognized as being efficient and adequate (Würgler *et al.*, 1975). In contrast, the problem of statistical analysis for dominant lethal mutation assays can not be considered solved, due to the uncertainties of the biological parameters (Krüger, 1971). The *reproducibility* of the results should first be ascertained.

In the past, results obtained with one material sometimes differed from year to year in the same laboratory, so much so as to produce contradictions. It is known that even in a homogeneous strain of the same mammalian species handled by the same researchers, results of experiments performed in different places can lead to partly or totally different conclusions. These differences, which in the context of classical toxicology can generally be immediately explained, can have unexpected consequences in the field of genetic toxicology. The confidence limits must be large. Consequently, experimental protocols should be rigorously standardized and the *reproducibility* of the test thoroughly controlled.

(4) To the requirements reviewed above, must be added another: This is the ability of the test to *fit* the greatest number of practical situations, and to detect the greatest number of mutation types. In Chapters 1 and 2, we have seen that some tests allow the mutation rate to be estimated for only one locus or, at the most, a few loci. Other tests deal with mutations of a specific chromosome, e.g. sex-linked mutations in *Drosophila*. Finally, other tests aim to investigate the chromosome damage as a whole, independent of the genetic consequences. No test is at present capable of evaluating the bulk of mutations induced by a given mutagen at a specific generation. Thus, a progressive battery of tests is required for each substance (suggestions in Chapter 10).

(5) Another quality of a reliable test is that it should be *rapidly* performed. As prompt an answer as possible is expected from the laboratory. If this requirement were not subordinated to the proceeding ones, it would suggest that lower organisms are to be preferred to the higher organisms. It is true that the majority of tests on mammals require months of work. From a practical point of view, however, the time necessary to perform a test should be proportionate to the importance of the problem to be solved. For example, the mutagenic power of alkylating agents occurring incidentally in the environment is sufficiently known, so that, for toxicological purposes, it is no longer necessary to spend much time in performing long-term assays in mammals, except for 'positive controls' in which such agents can be used.

In contrast, many critical substances, real sources of trouble, certainly deserve long-term study in mammals. In these cases, it is the only way to proceed for assessing the precise risks for man.

(6) Finally, there are two non-negligible qualities of a test: to be *easy* to perform and to be *inexpensive*. To be really efficient, a test should become almost routine.

However, most tests require a thorough scientific training, far beyond the practice of traditional toxicology. Therefore, it is prudent to select the methods adapted to the trained personnel available. It is obvious that cost is a limiting factor. How is one to reproduce experiments requiring tens of thousands of mammals in experiments dealing with just one chemical, and then to extend the test to hundreds of chemicals?

EVALUATION OF THE TESTS: ADVANTAGES AND DISADVANTAGES

On the basis of the preceding requirements, we can try to evaluate the tests briefly described in Chapters 1 and 2.

Experiments with micro-organisms have the advantage of being easy and quick. They are more readily suited to statistical analysis of large samples, and are, in this respect, more precise. However, they generally deal with only one locus, or at most a few loci. In other words, they are concerned with a very small portion of the genome (e.g. the gene *histidine* of *Salmonella*, *ad 3* of

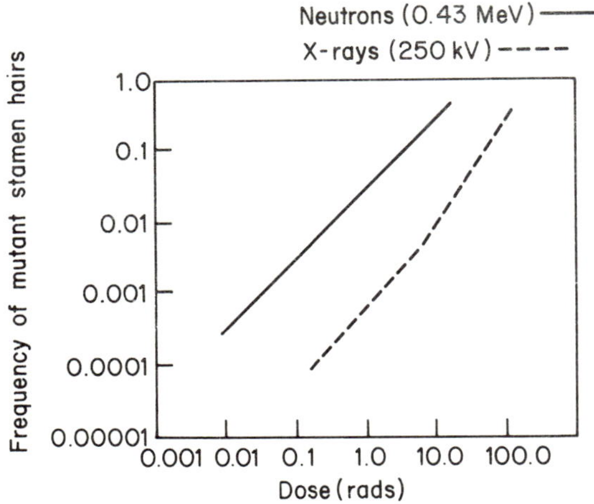

FIG. 19. Comparison of the effects of monoenergetic fast neutrons and X-rays on the frequency of anthocyanic mutants induced in *Tradescantia* stamen hairs (Sparrow *et al.*, 1972)

Neurospora, ad 7 of *Schizosaccharomyces)* which may react in a particular way compared with other loci. In this respect, a specific locus can also be exceptionally resistant to a given mutagenic agent. This abnormal resistance decreases the scope of the test considerably, since no generalization of the results to the whole genome is possible.

Genetic tests dealing with cells of higher plant organs cultured *in vitro* or whole plants *in vivo* have the advantage of allowing good cytological observations. Some of these tests are very sensitive (e.g. anthocyanic mutants of *Tradescantia*, as developed by Sparrow and coworkers, which allowed in particular cosmic rays to be detected in biosatellites). With this biological material, the effects of doses as low as 0.1 R of X-rays and 0.01 R of fast neutrons (Sparrow *et al.*, 1972) (Fig. 19) can be detected.

Unfortunately, *Tradescantia* cells are less suitable for studying the effects of chemicals, due to the low permeability to many compounds. Variable responses to toxic agents strongly restrict the scope of these tests.

Another plant test as sensitive as the previous one makes use of biochemical mutants such as *waxy* in pollen grains of Gramineae (Chapter 1). This kind of test allowed investigation of the effects of very low doses of γ-rays and the risk of radiation from ^{90}r (Ehrenberg and Eriksson, 1966). It is also applicable to low doses of chemicals (Sulovska *et al.*, 1969). However, although the results obtained with plants are of major interest in studying modifications of the biosphere following various pollutions (Chapter 9), the possibility of extrapolation to man is questionable. This can be explained, among other things, by the special sensitivity or resistance of plant cells, and also by metabolic differences.

Tests of group III which investigate the effects directly visible at the chromosome level have the advantage of rapidity and efficiency. However, sensitivity is sometimes reduced by the occurrence of a relatively high frequency of spontaneous chromosomal aberrations even under strictly controlled experimental conditions. Spontaneous lesions can be particularly numerous in cultured animal cells. We mentioned previously the fact that the standardized use of plant tissue cultures is not very feasible because of the existence of interfering endogenous factors, including endoploidization which destabilize the cultures. Another difficulty of these tests arises from the lack of synchrony, or from the poor possibility of synchronization of cell divisions. This is the case for roots in the plant kingdom, but also for several animal tissues cultured *in vitro*. Finally, it is not possible to foresee the exact genetic consequences of the chromosomal damage observed.

In Chapter 2 we outlined a tentative classification of chromosomal lesions as a function of their most probable remote genetic consequences rather than as a single criterion designed to evaluate cytotoxicity.

The micronucleus test and sister-chromatid exchange test have been considered interesting alternatives for detecting chromosome damage and repair. The first does not require special training in cytology, and is relatively easy, rapid and inexpensive.

Contrary to the analysis of chromosome damage in metaphases, it does not readily allow quantitative evaluation for the following reasons. First, as already mentioned, a certain (unknown) proportion of micronuclei is incorporated in the main nuclei; inversely, some micronuclei are expelled from the erythroblast, thus escaping microscopic detection in both cases. Secondly, small micronuclei corresponding to minutes (small chromosome fragments), more likely to result in genetic modifications can be prematurely resorbed in the cytoplasm, thereby becoming indistinguishable. The resorption kinetics of micronuclei have previously been investigated in plant cells (Moutschen and Moutschen-Dahmen, 1958). In mammals, the kinetics are certainly quite different. Thirdly, modificiations of the kinetics of the investigated cell population can be induced by many toxic agents, at least at high doses. Such modifications of mitotic cycles should be pretested for each agent. Fourthly, a large proportion of important chromosome lesions, e.g. symmetrical translocations, do not result in losses of parts of chromosomes and remain undetected. We insisted on the fact that such rearrangements have a much greater risk of being inherited.

With regards to sister-chromatid exchanges, although there is a reasonable presumption that they are due to DNA breakage and reunion, the exact relationship between these modifications and DNA repair at the molecular level in both mutagenesis and carcinogenesis is still poorly understood. More confusing is the fact that the dose–effect relationship is generally only relevant within a small range of doses, even after treatment with powerful mutagens such as ionizing radiations where the curve rapidly reaches a plateau (review in Wolff, 1977, and Evans, 1977). This 'saturation effect' should be analysed for each agent tested. In spite of the misleading possibilities, these two alternatives can be considered valuable ancillary tests in chromosome breakage analysis. In some cases, they could also serve as screening tests to pilot time-consuming cytological analyses.

The genetic effects can in fact be more fully estimated in whole organisms, especially in *Drosophila* or mammals like mouse.

If, in *Drosophila,* no test allows the investigation of all types of mutations, these tests are concerned with a portion of the genome incomparably larger than in lower organisms. Some tests allow the analysis of the majority of mutations in about one-fifth of the genome. According to Abrahamson *et al.* (1980), the Muller-5 test can deal with 830 potentially lethal mutations. It can partly cope with the difficulty of performing the experiments on a very large scale as in lower organisms. Although it is necessary to obtain successive generations, such tests can provide answers within a relatively short time. However, there is a long distance to cover between the fly and man!

In the mouse, we described a number of ingenious methods for dealing with specific loci. In the past, they yielded important information on the genetic effects of ionizing radiations and alkylating agents. These experiments require such large numbers of animals, however, that no laboratory in the world could possibly think seriously of carrying out such tests systematically. Moreover, besides the long time required to obtain conclusive results, these tests analyse but a tiny part of the genetic system for only one class of mutations: recessive visible (with the additional possibility of detecting the dominant visible mutations*).

Because of the difficulties involved in long-term tests and large sample experiments, so-called spot tests have been worked out in mammals. Since in the classical spot test (Chapter 2), a large number of cells per animal are treated; large numbers of animals are not required as in the seven-locus test. This test is considered to be sensitive since each spot corresponds to a mutagenic event. Besides genetic effects, teratogenic aberrations and potential carcinogenic effects can be detected. There are, however, some discrepancies in the classification of the spots which result in some confusion, particularly with weak mutagens. Standardization is needed. Moreover, it is obvious that some spots are not of genetic origin. Finally, with the spot test, the possibility of the test substance of crossing the placental barrier should be known. Examination of sperm abnormalities has been suggested as a simple test in various mammals. The observation of sperm abnormalities is certainly easy and quick, technically speaking, but it is clear that an unknown number of modifications of sperm shape or stainability are not of genetic origin. To increase the specificity of this so-called sperm test, mutants deficient in acrosome components such as pronase or hyaluronidase or some specific antigens have been used (Moutschen and Colizzi, 1975). This will probably improve the possibility of scoring the real genetic damage, either spontaneous or induced, but at the present stage such investigations should be considered ancillary to the more elaborate methods in mammals, except perhaps for occupational investigations of human populations where they can yield interesting information.

* In recent years, a valuable method for detecting dominant cataract mutations in mice has been worked out (Kratochvilova and Ehling, 1979; Kratochvilova, 1981). It is sensitive for testing ^{137}Cs γ-rays. It will be an interesting alternative test system in the future.

Dominant lethal mutation assays in mouse, slightly modified in a few other mammals, are generally considered convenient. However, they are handicapped by the occurrence of a somewhat large proportion of embryos degenerating spontaneously. Even when it is possible to avoid some mistakes such as those arising from a high level of inbreeding in the strains utilized, it is not generally possible to minimize the spontaneous background of mutations below a certain baseline level. Therefore, to be efficient, these tests should be performed on a large number of animals.

Finally, these tests give only a gross estimation of various classes of mutations of different nature, some being point mutations with minor damage, and some corresponding to major chromsomal damage.

Tests that aim to investigate chromosome non-disjunctions or sex-linked recessive lethal mutations in mammals are in general not yet sufficiently worked out to evaluate accurately their predictability. Chromosome non-disjunctions still remain a real problem. Except in plants where observation is easy, their detection is more problematic in other organisms such as mammals, as in the method mentioned above. Simpler and inexpensive methods such as the observation of extra Y chromosomes in sperm have been worked out. This biased method leaves the problem largely unsolved for the following reasons: only one chromosome of the genome is concerned which is far from being a large proportion in mammals; non-disjunction is exclusively analysed in males, whereas it is well known that an important proportion of diseases in which a trisomic chromosome is observed arises also from females.

Methods in which mammals are used as intermediates — the host-mediated assays — have in common some advantages and some non negligible disadvantages. Since the organism tested is actually a lower organism, they have the advantages of the methods applicable to such organisms, especially rapidity and to some extent efficiency. These tests allow one to check how a mutagenic compound is detoxified by the mammalian system, and thus to estimate the reactions of defence against deleterious agents. Conversely, they allow one to detect if chemicals found to be inactive *in vitro* are transformed into real mutagens *in vivo,* from which a better assessment of the risks for man can be inferred (Chapter 7).

In the first protocol, these tests can not be accepted as such. Firstly, lower organisms are not always devoid of pathogenic properties. They can continue to grow in biological fluids after being injected, and their metabolic activity is maintained during the test period. Consequently, the sample in which the mutagenic activity is measured is very likely to differ, sometimes markedly, from the sample that received the mutagenic agent at the beginning of the treatment. The metabolic state of the micro-organism capable of being modified by the mammalian environment is therefore scarcely controlled. Furthermore, micro-organisms, even those with a slowly metabolic turnover such as *Neurospora* conidia, can give rise to secondary undesirable reactions in the mammal.

Secondly, the complement present in the serum of mammals can also interact in micro-organism mutagenesis. It might be activated by natural antibodies against various micro-organisms. Some compounds diffusing from micro-organisms can also activate the C_3 fraction of the complement even in the absence of antigen–antibody reactions involving the pre-existence of natual antibodies. Such immunological reactions should be known in each specific case before performing the host-mediated assay.

Another difficulty arises from the fact that the metabolic processes of the micro-organism can partly or even totally inactivate mutagens with or without detoxification by the host cells. Conversely, micro-organisms can activate metabolites normally inactive in mammalian cells into dangerous mutagens (Chapter 9).

As stated by Fishbein *et al.* (1970, in Gen. Refs.) (and restated since on the basis of the results of numerous experiments on repair processes as reported in Chapter 6), it should be kept in mind that repair processes in micro-organisms differ from those occurring in mammalian cells. In an environment as unusual for *Neurospora* conidia as mammalian body fluids, repair processes of micro-organisms can also be greatly altered. Finally, repair processes of the host can possibly be influenced by the micro-organism itself. The location of the micro-organism in the body is of importance, particularly in relation to blood circulation in the liver. The systematic recovery of micro-organisms from the same site in the body could result in a selection of mutants leading to a false idea of the real mutagenic potentiality of the substance under test. This selection of mutants can modify the mutagenic spectrum especially when genetic damage is lethal in micro-organisms but not or to a lesser extent in the host cells, possibly because of the better bufferring of higher organisms. Also the elimination of a certain proportion of cells will depend entirely on strong modifications of the structure of the micro-organism population. Finally, extrapolation of the data obtained with host-mediated assays at low doses of chemicals still appears difficult. To facilitate this extrapolation, it was proposed to replace the micro-organisms by mammalian or even human cells from *in vitro* cultures. This method would give a considerable amount of information on detoxification processes. However, all the problems mentioned above should previously have been solved.

SOME REFLECTIONS

From the preceding discussion, it appears that no mutagenicity test now available has all the qualities previously required. There is no particular method that permits all types of mutations to be detected simultaneously and even less other possible genetic effects, e.g. convertogenic and recombinogenic effects. Thus, at the present stage, it is essential to work out different tests to enable a sufficiently large amount of data to be collected. Some strategies will be proposed in Chapter 10. We stated before that to allow a more direct extrapolation of the data to man, tests on mammals have been favoured. Reactions to toxic substances are greatly influenced by genetic background, not only in man but also in laboratory animals. These variations depend on the species, sex or even the individual animal. A difference as small as one pair of genes can sometimes increase sensitivity or, inversely, resistance to toxic substances. These differences, well known in classical toxicology, are also valid for genetic effects. The systematic study of such differences, their causes and mechanisms is the main objective of experimental pharmacogenetics (Meier, 1963, in Gen. Refs.; Evans, 1982).

Knowledge of these differences should in principle permit the real sensitivity towards a substance to be ascertained and to determine whether this sensitivity is abnormally increased or reduced.

It should be pointed out that in the large majority of experiments on mammals, males have been tested exclusively, because the successive stages of spermatogenesis are well known. Moreover, males generally show more regular responses to mutagenic agents than females. This model in which only males are treated is therefore oversimplified.

The routes of treatment do not often correspond with the reality of the human environment. Thus, it is considered to be more accurate and efficient to treat animals by intraperitoneal or intravenous injection with substances to which man is ordinarily only exposed through the digestive or respiratory system. In fact, this procedure does not allow the real risks to be assessed, but leads either to an overestimation or an underestimation of the effects. This is the case of substances such ethylene oxide, propylene oxide, chlorhydrin, epichlorhydrin, etc. (Chapters 4, 5 and 7).

In a detailed piece of research, Ehrenberg *et al.* (1974) attempted to evaluate the genetic hazards of ethylene oxide by submitting mice to gaseous mixtures containing increased quantities of this toxic substance. Although difficult to achieve with precision, such types of experiments should be extended to a larger number of substances to which man is only exposed in gaseous phase.

Contaminants are sometimes mutagenic or even toxic for bacterial cells to a greater extent than for human cells, as in the case of antibiotics, and unpredicted modifications of the intestinal flora due to bacterial mutations can generate problems. Extremely virulent strains of mutant bacteria can proliferate as well.

The control of intestinal bacteria has found practical application. Mutated bacterial strains can acquire the ability to activate ineffective promutagenic substances into mutagens. Conversely, intestinal bacteria can contribute to the detoxification of dangerous drugs. The importance of these modifications in bacterial populations should be kept in mind for the surveillance and monitoring of human populations by analysis of body fluids (Chapter 9).

If the results obtained with plant cells can scarcely be extrapolated to man, they have quite different applications in other fields. Plants systems are valuable in detecting the potential mutagenicity of environmental pollutants. It would be convenient to master sensitive biological systems to reveal cytogenetic effects in the environment and to locate pollution periods. For example, in *Tradescantia* stamen hairs, Sparrow *et al.* (1972) detected abnormalities induced by an accidental contamination of which nobody was aware. This pollutant was later identified (see Schairer *et al.*, 1980a, b, in Chapter 8). On the basis of data collected on the effects of pollutants on plant cells, we suggested as suitable material, antheridial threads of the alga *Chara* which is sensitive and has relatively large chromosomes (Moutschen and Moutschen-Dahmen, 1971). In this plant, a test system akin to the micronucleus test in mammals could be developed with the advantage that the kinetics of the cell populations of antheridia can be controlled. This test system is unfortunately restricted to water pollution.

Recently, ferns including the royal fern (*Osmunda regalis*) were adopted as biological material for bioassays of mutagens *in situ,* i.e. for revealing mutations induced by pollutants in populations, thus helping to identify potential genotoxic agents. This material has been successfully applied to aquatic ecosystems (review in Klekowski, 1978). *Osmunda* spores and prothallae in fact were previously used to investigate the effects of ionizing radiations (Howard and Haigh, 1968) and of a bifunctional alkylating agent, Myleran (Moutschen, 1962).

Such experimental research designed to detect genotoxic pollutants of the biosphere is still in its infancy. Knowledge of the genetics of such materials should certainly be increased. On the other hand, the exact level of spontaneous mutations or chromosome damage in non-polluted populations should first be investigated. More sensitive indicators of mutagenic pollutants not only in water but also in atmospheric systems should be worked out, for instance, in higher plants. In fact, in the past, morphological modifications of wild and cultivated plants allowed gross pollutions to be detected. This methodology, if improved, will have a bright future (see Chapter 9).

Besides already well-tested systems, often too insensitive, one wonders if it would not also be appropriate to work out new test systems. Experiments on mammals closer to man such as simians could be considered. However, our genetic knowledge of these animals is still quite scanty. It would require years of work and great expense to obtain sufficient background data. The marmoset has been used to measure the frequency of aneuploid mutations (Bobrow and Ejiwunmi, 1978), but a few biological peculiarities of this material should be specified. *Tupaia* is another attractive biological system often suggested for experiments on mutations.

Since their metabolic pathways resemble more closely those of man, simians could also be selected in host-mediated assays to investigate the detoxification of chemical mutagens. These genetic tests could be complemented with detailed biochemical studies especially with labelled compounds such as tritium or ^{14}C. This kind of chemical research was previously performed with powerful mutagenic alkylating agents (Ross, 1962, in Gen. Refs.), but should be extended to all compounds suspected of mutagenicity. There are also perhaps ethical restrictions to using primates in such experiments. Because of the difficulties involved in using these animals on a large scale, it would be more appropriate to develop multipurpose tests in rodents, particularly mouse.

We have already mentioned the advantages of simultaneous investigations of all sex-linked mutations and of chromosome breakage in mouse. For measuring the effects of chronic exposure to environmental pollutants, these tests should ideally cover successive generations.

The development of immunological methods designed to detect rare biochemical cell mutants is certainly progressing fast. They have the advantage of efficiency, and often the results can be submitted to simple and automated statistics. Being short-term methods, they save time and money, and allow a greater number of potentially mutagenic substances to be tested. Also, they are applicable at two distinct levels: first, in experimental test systems, and second, directly in man for monitoring populations after chronic exposures to mutagens or in cases of acute accidents (Chapter 9). Malling (1981) made some interesting statements about the possibility of extrapolation of data from mammals to man for risk assessment. In experimental animals, the frequency of rare mutant cells (e.g. for an abnormal haemoglobin) should be correlated with the frequency of such mutations hereditarily transmitted at the first generation of treated animals. The second step would be to correlate the frequency of the selected mutation in an animal with the frequency of the same mutation in man, taking into account pharmacological differences.

Two important questions arise, however: (1) In the experiments, genes are selected not only for technical convenience, but also because they are common to both man and mammals. This selection gives great specificity to the test. It means that these genes have shown a great stability during the evolution of mammals. Now, it should be kept in mind that differences of mutability between loci exist as demonstrated in the Russel test after exposure to ionizing radiations (Russel, 1951). Categories of not-so-stable genes, specific to humans and showing greater mutability might exist. Such genes would therefore escape the investigation, because of not being their equivalent in animal populations. (2) As already mentioned in Chapter 2, there is the necessity of automating the procedure. Since the mutations investigated are rare, sometimes very rare, events, their recording is time-consuming.

Besides the gross mutations previously mentioned, the possible occurrence of less conspicuous mutational events, e.g. modifying quantitative characters, should not be omitted in the test battery. Such mutations could influence, for example, the size and the weight of organs, the ratio between parts of the body, the amount of secreted substances, etc. They are not, properly speaking, defects, i.e. deleterious effects in the genetic system due to a major mutation. They are minor mutations, and their effects on the phenotype are far from being always visible. It is known that quantitative characters are controlled by more than one gene, therefore being polygenic in nature, and inherited in a particular manner. It has been demonstrated (e.g. Mather, 1949; Dobzhansky, 1957; Wright, 1968, in Gen. Refs.) that when occurring frequently these quantitative mutations can be of high significance for the evolution of genetic systems. At present it is not well established that quantitative mutations result in beneficial or deleterious effects, especially within a short period, although there is a reasonable guess that some human diseases are inherited that way (Fraser, 1981). This problem is certainly at a level of complexity far beyond the problems commonly found in genetic toxicology.

Concerning induced quantitative mutations, the data available are very scanty, and this aspect of mutagenesis is now added to the programme of future methodology (review in Ramel, 1983).

Finally, it is of great importance to know if all possible genetic effects have actually been covered by the battery of tests described. We are still forced to answer this question in the negative. In this context, mutations corresponding to gain or loss of chromosomes have not been systmetically sought. Systematic tests of chromosome non-disjunction could also be worked out (Chapter 2).

Another point worth mentioning is the possibility for certain mutagenic agents to modify the crossing-over frequency (recombinogenic effect). This is the case for the male of *Drosophila,* where it is normally absent but can be induced by ionizing radiations. This occurs in the little fish, guppy *Lebistes reticulatus*, a possible model for such studies. These modifications can have important long-term consequences. In fact, each living being in equilibrium with its environment shows an optimized recombination rate. All modifications of this somewhat delicate internal equilibrium can disturb the variability potential of a species and possibly its adaptability. Too abrupt perturbations of the recombination mechanisms could in the end be more important for a population than some deleterious mutations which could be eventually eliminated.

It was also reported in the literature that some mutagenic agents can induce or modify such phenomena as conversion and paramutation (Brink, 1958). Increasingly tests on several organisms, e.g. yeasts, include conversion tests performed at the same time as the more classical tests of mutations (Chapter 1). The origin of paramutations, mainly investigated in higher plants (Brink, 1958), is still too obscure to be debated at length here, but nobody knows about the long-term consequences of modifications of this kind.

From the arguments briefly discussed in this chapter, it is clear that mutagenic effects of substances found in the environment are far from being the only possible genetic effects. Therefore, in the future, a battery of tests should be introduced which detects all potential genetic effects.

Chapter 4

The Search For Mutagens in the Environment

'Tout s'élève contre eux; les beautez (*sic*) de Nature
Que leur rage troubla de venin et d'ordure
Se confondent en mire et se lèvent contre eux'

Agrippa d'Augibné
Les Maudits

Historically, geneticists tried to investigate the mutagenic effect of ionizing radiations before the effects of chemicals. Arguably this priority might justify one chapter being devoted to genetic hazards of atomic energy, but, as stated by Crow (quoted in Sanders, 1969), 'To consider only radiation hazards may be to ignore the submerged part of the iceberg.' This statement justifies the other chapters.

Since the pioneer research of Auerbach and Robson (1944, 1947), Auerbach, *et al.* (1947), Rapoport (1946, 1948), and Auerbach (1949) in the animal kingdom, of Gustafsson and MacKey (1948) in the plant kingdom, and the outburst of chemical mutagenesis, geneticists became aware of the potential hazards of many substances occurring in the environment. Could it not be that a substance found to be of little or no toxicity by the usual methods shows a high mutagenicity in man?

The number of chemicals used by man is enormous. More than 500 new compounds flood the market every year, swelling the mass of thousands already available. In the two preceding chapters, it was stated that a complete study of a compound for mutagenicity requires a considerable array of techniques (see also Chapter 10), and it would be unrealistic to investigate in detail the mutagenicity of all potentially mutagenic compounds.

Two main questions arise: Where in the environment are the mutagenic substances located? and How can they be detected and the risks evaluated?

We propose a general classification of the substances into three groups according to the way in which they occur in the environment (Table 1). This classification involves a correlation between the amount of the substance in the environment and the risks for man.

TABLE 1. Classification of environmental mutagens

Group I. Mutagenic substances synthesized by man and used directly in specific conditions

- A. Pharmaceuticals
  - a. antitumour agents
  - b. antibiotics
  - c. narcotics
  - d. contraceptives
  - e. excipients
  - f. anaesthetics
- B. Pesticides
  - a. insecticides
  - b. raticides
  - c. herbicides
  - d. fungicides
  - e. molluscicides
  - f. nematocides
- C. Additives
  - a. food
  - b. other (cosmetics)
- D. Biological contaminants

Group II. Mutagenic substances used in industry or occurring in the environment as by-products of industry

- A. Industrial alkylating agents
- B. Organic solvents organo- metallic compounds
- C. Water pollutants
- D. Air pollutants
- E. Heavy metals

Group III. Natural mutagenic substances

- A. Alkaloids
- B. Products of microbial metabolism

GROUP I: MUTAGENS EXTRACTED OR SYNTHESIZED BY MAN AND USED DIRECTLY IN SPECIFIC CONDITIONS

Pharmaceuticals

In 1980, a symposium was held in Paris with the purpose of issuing some guidelines for mutagenicity testing of new drugs on the basis of recommendations by the Committee on Proprietary Medicinal Products (1979) (Draper and Griffin, 1980). A general conclusion emerged that 'a minimum package' of tests should be performed for each new drug, but with some flexibility, leaving to the manufacturer the possibility of selecting alternative experimental models. For drugs already marketed the conclusion is far less clear. In fact, this statement reflects the diversity which exists in the field of pharmaceuticals. For this reason we selected several categories of drugs under different headings according to their different genetic implications.

(1) Antitumour agents

Since the discovery of the tremendous mutagenic potential of the majority of antitumour agents, geneticists still continue to test repeatedly these molecules, particularly alkylating agents, in all possible biological systems.

Now, the circumstances in which these chemicals are used are relatively rare and the risks well defined and generally accepted. The main application of these chemicals is in the therapeutics of malignant tumours. Generally, the treatment of seriously ill patients with these mutagenic agents is not an important genetic problem. We should just make a restriction in a few cases. Firstly, in non-malignant tumours, irradiation with ionizing radiations or treatment with drugs can cause a significant dose genetically to be administered. Secondly, in diseases such as Hodgkin's disease, in which long-term treatment can be a grave risk for the progeny of the patients, *Vinca rosea* alkaloids have been used as an adjuvant therapy. Experiments designed to demonstrate mutagenicity of these alkaloids yielded negative results (review in Degraeve, 1978). They should be preferred to far more mutagenic treatments whenever possible.

An interesting antineoplastic compound, *cis*-diamminedichloroplatinum, showed positive mutagenic responses in bacteria (Andersen, 1979; Beck and Fisch, 1980) and in Chinese hamster V79 cells (Zwelling *et al.*, 1979). This compound is clastogenic in haemopoietic tissues *in vivo* and induces sister-chromatid exchanges *in vitro* in human and rabbit cells (Morrison *et al.*, 1981).

It was suspected that mutagenicity could be at least partly due to impurities or degradation products. However, new data indicate only a weak effect of the degradation complexes in bacteria (Peer and Litz, 1981). If confirmed with other test systems the properties of this class of compounds could be suitably exploited in therapeutics.

In all these cases, the consequences of treatment at the population level are

TABLE 2. Genetic effects of some antibiotics used as antitumour drugs in higher organisms

Substance	Material	Criteria	Authors
Azaserine	*Tradescantia paludosa* root tips	Chromosomal aberrations	Tanaka and Sigimura, 1956
	Human cells	Chromosomal aberrations	Biesele, 1958
	Drosophila melanogaster	Gonad mosaicism	Altenburg and Browning, 1964
	Vicia faba root tips	Chromosomal aberrations	Kihlman, 1964; Davidson, 1965
Mitomycin C	*Vicia faba* root tips	Chromosomal aberrations	Merz, 1961
	Human leucocytes	Chromosomal aberrations and mitotic inhibitions	Nowell, 1964
		Chromosomal aberrations	Cohen and Shaw, 1964; Shaw and Cohen, 1965
	Dropsophila melanogaster	Sister-chromatid exchanges	Morad *et al.*, 1973
		Crossing-over modifications	Latt, 1974; Suzuki, 1965
		Recessive lethal mutations	Mukherjee, 1965
	Habrobracon	Dominant lethal mutations	Smith, 1969
Streptomycin	*Salmonella typhimurium*	Host-mediated assay Ratio prototrophs/auxotrophs	Gabridge *et al.*, 1963
Streptonigrin	Human leucocytes	Chromosomal aberrations	Cohen *et al.*, 1963
	Vicia faba root tip	Chromosomal aberrations	Kihlman, 1964; Kihlman and Odmark, 1965
	Mammalian cells (*in vitro*)	Chromosomal aberrations and mitotic anomalies	Puck, 1964
	Mouse ovaries	Meiotic aberrations	Jagiello, 1967
Daunomycin	Human leucocytes	Chromosomal aberrations	Vig *et al.*, 1968a, b, 1969; Vig, 1971a
Adriamycin	Human leucocytes	Chromosomal aberrations	Vig, 1971b
	Human leucocytes	Chromosomal aberrations	Perry and Evans, 1975
Bleomycin	Human leucocytes	Chromosomal aberrations	Ohama, and Kadotani, 1970
	Bone marrow of patients	Chromosomal aberrations	Bornstein *et al.*, 1971
	Nigella damascena seeds	Chromosomal aberrations	Moutschen, *et al.*, 1973a
Phleomycin	*Vicia faba* root tip	Chromosomal aberrations	Mattingly, 1967
		Chromosomal aberrations	Kihlman *et al.*, 1967
	Mouse ovaries	Meiotic aberrations	Jagiello, 1868
	Human leucocytes	Chromosomal aberrations	Jacobs *et al.*, 1969

quite low because only a few patients are treated. This is not the case for alkylating agents when they are components of pesticides or when they belong to group II. Their effects will be surveyed later.

(2) Antibiotics (including antifungal, antiprotozoan and anthelminthic substances)

Antibiotics that show a high mutagenic effect in mammalian cells generally belong to the class of antitumour substances. Consequently, the risks are the same as those of alkylating agents acting in the same circumstances (for mitomycin C, actinomycin, daunomycin and adriamycin, see review in Vig, 1977).

It is not unlikely that antibiotics other than those indicated in Table 2 induce mutagenic effects, but few data are as yet available. The case of isoniazid, which is thought to produce metabolically the well-known mutagen, hydrazine, will be discussed in Chapter 7 as an experimental model in genetic toxicology.

However, even though the mutagenic effects of antibiotics have been demonstrated in various test systems, the question of their use should be objectively considered in view of important risk–benefit considerations. In fact, it should be kept in mind that, as a rule, these substances are given to acute cases but generally for short periods of time. From another point of view, there is a definite possibility of antibiotics modifying bacterial populations in the intestinal human flora, by mutation or selection in a way detrimental to man. On the other hand, the fact that some antibiotics increase the mutagenic effects of some compounds should be taken into account. This is the case of chloramphenicol as well as with some other broad-spectrum antibiotics.

Other antibiotic or antiparasitic drugs also raise some problems, due to their activation into real mutagens by intestinal microbial flora. This is the case of the antiparasitic drug 4-isothiocyano-4′-nitrodiphenylamine which is not mutagenic in *in vitro* systems with or without liver homogenates but becomes activated by gut bacteria into an ultimate mutagen recovered in the urine (Batzinger *et al.*, 1978). Such examples are not uncommon. Body fluids such as urine and bile can also activate promutagens, including pharmaceuticals, into ultimate mutagens (details in Chapter 9).

In fact, all antibiotics which, one way or another markedly modify or even annihilate the intestinal flora, will cause similar problems.

Some antiprotozoan and anthelminthic substances are also potential hazards. In this respect, we can mention ethidium chloride, ethidium bromide, 8-hydroxyquinoline, and especially a series of antischistosomal substances derived from 10-thioxanthenone such as 1-[[2-(diethylamino)ethyl]amino]-4-methylthioxanthen-a-one (Miracil-D, lucanthone).

The effects of such substances vary from one species to another or even show great individual variations. An organophosphorus pesticide, trichlorfon (metrifonate), has a special position. It is used not only in insecticide mixtures but also as an anthelminthic, sometimes at fairly high doses. The question of whether it is first metabolized into another organophosphorus compound is still debated. The cytogenetic effects of these substances in the mouse have been reviewed (Moutschen *et al.*, 1981). Such activity has only been demonstrated at doses much higher than those utilized for therapeutic effects and those incorporated in insecticides. The effect is also strongly dependent on the test system.

(3) Narcotics and related substances

Above and beyond the genetic problems caused by the use of therapeutic alkylating agents, the use and abuse of narcotics is at a higher level of complexity. If it is demonstrated that some molecules of the morphine group induce chromosomal aberrations (Camara and Angulo-Carpio, 1949; Oehlkers, 1953; Scheibe, 1959; Gilmour *et al.*, 1971; Falek *et al.*, 1972) in various genetic systems, it is difficult to imagine the future of a human population completely addicted to these drugs, apart from all the genetic considerations!

The appearance of lysergic acid diethylamide (LSD) raises more complicated problems of control since this hallucinogen can be more easily and widely spread. Data about its genetic effects are still contradictory. On the one hand some researchers (Irwin and Egozcue, 1967; Cohen *et al.*, 1967a, b; Jarvik and Kato, 1968, etc.) found clastogenic properties in human cells *in vitro* and *in vivo*. On the other hand, no chromosome abnormalities were observed in persons suffering from LSD addiction (Loughman *et al.*, 1967; Sparkes *et al.*, 1968; Bender and Sankar, 1968). Whereas Browning (1968) and Vann (1969) mentioned mutations in *Drosophila,* Grace *et al.* (1968) failed to detect any effect in the same organism; Zetterberg (1969) reported negative results in the fungus *Ophiostoma*. Whatever the meaning of these results, the clastogenic and mutagenic effects of LSD do not deserve the unremitting attention of geneticists since the real problems clearly lie elsewhere.

Other psychotropic drugs have also been tested for potential mutagenicity. Amphetamine sulphate and related compounds have a strong effect on segmentation-division of the newt (Sentein, 1962). Clastogenicity in mammalian cultured cells by phenothiazine (Gilmour *et al.*, 1971), chlorpromazine and perphenazine (Nielsen *et al.*, 1968) has been demonstrated. A completely unrelated compound, psilocybine (Eberle and Leuner, 1970), is clastogenic in treated patients. Except in these latter experiments no mutagenic tests were performed on mammals *in toto*.

Some inhalational anaesthetics have also been tested, including trichloroethylene and to a lesser extent fluorene, vinyl ether, halothane, cyclopropane and nitrous oxide (Baden and Simmon, 1980). Some of them yielded highly positive results in *Drosophila* and *Tradescantia* stamen hairs. However, due to the short duration of exposure under modern conditions of anaesthesia, genetic effects from such substances are not likely to occur in man.

The conclusion of the present section is that, before releasing substances onto the market the risk–benefits balance should be carefully checked. The genetic problem is just one aspect of a tremendous unsolved problem. There is still room here for multiple investigations.

(4) Contraceptives

As in the case of other substances, the potential mutagenicity of contraceptives deserved the attention of researchers although the results are still somewhat scanty. Carr (1967) observed chromosomal lesions in women taking oral contraceptives, but more recent reports (Bishun *et al.*, 1973, 1976) from observations of women submitted to classical hormonal contraceptives found no significant differences between treated women and controls. Combinations of three progestagens and two oestrogens gave negative results in *Drosophila* in a sex-linked, recessive lethal mutation test (Parádi, 1981). Such experimental results can hardly be extrapolated to man.

The fact that these compounds are generally administered for a long period prompts caution, since our knowledge of the cumulative effects of these substances is still indecisive. Bishun *et al.* (1976) insist on the difficulty of establishing causal relations for long-term treatment, especially since the components of contraceptives are continuously changing both qualitatively and quantitatively.

In another quite remote class of contraceptive substances, prostaglandins also have other therapeutic uses. They are known to induce chromosome damage in plant cells (Moutschen *et al.*, 1973b). However, these effects have not been demonstrated in *in vivo* mammalian systems in which few long-term experiments have been carried out. Further research should be based on metabolic studies attempting to prove that these substances are quite adequately and rapidly detoxified. Other consequences of the use of contraceptives are beyond the scope of mutagenesis. Although contraceptives are undoubtedly an efficient means of controlling over-population, they appear able in the long run to modify the genetic structure of human populations. These modifications should not be accepted without a carefully controlled investigation by competent geneticists. This generalized practice would lead to substitution of a completely artificial mechanism of selection within the process of natural selection, a situation wrought with danger. At the beginning of the century, Galton and Haldane already realized that selection as it occurs in human populations leads to a decreased frequency of various social characters considered desirable to man, such as, for instance, intelligence. It was precisely one of the aims of Galton's eugenics, based among other things on statistical considerations, to try to reverse this tendency. Selection pressure, blindly and preferentially applied to a specific group of individuals, can lead to disaster. Before organizing massive contraception, it would be imperative to define the genetic load of the population under investigation. However, the search for adequate means of solving these multiple problems is really beyond the scope of genetic toxicology.

Pesticides

(insecticides, nematocides, molluscicides, raticides, herbicides and fungicides)

Various problems dealing with the mutagenicity of pesticides have been reviewed by Epstein and Legator (1971, in Gen. Refs.) and Moutschen (1979). More than 400 pesticides belonging to diverse chemical classes have been described, but only a relatively small proportion of these molecules have been tested and generally in a few short-term systems. Pesticides are widespread in the environment. DDT was even detected in the blood of auks living on remote islands, and modern insecticidal preparations such as aldrin, carbaryl, diazinon and malathion are certainly not less dangerous (Chapters 7 and 9).

A comprehensive review of pesticides would require a specialized text-book. Beside the obvious genetic and carcinogenic risks of some pesticides for man, there is another potentially even more important genetic hazard. This is the risk of upsetting the natural equilibrium of large populations, thereby generating secondary effects possibly more important than mutagenic effects. Ecological and genetic aspects of the problems are closely related. This is why it is worthwhile considering them together (see chapter 9).

Epstein and Legator (1971, in Gen. Refs.) classified pesticides logically. They distinguish (Fig. 20) (1) those that react mainly with DNA, and (2) those that react incidentally with DNA but without altering its structure, or which can inhibit some enzymatic reactions with indirect, but potentially significant, consequences.

In the first group, tests of mutagenicity in higher organisms might be somewhat limited though often experiments yielding positive results have been performed for entirely different reasons. On the other hand, in the second group, the potential mutagenicity of the compounds is often based on assumptions. Therefore such substances would require more extensive mutagenicity testing, particularly in higher organisms.

(1) Alkylating agents

In the class of the alkylating agents, epoxides are among the most used (Chapter 5). Ethylene imines such as apholate, TEPA and derivatives, and sulphates such as Aramite should also be mentioned.

Much research has involved investigations of reactions of alkylating agents with cell components, particularly DNA (review of the chemistry of alkylating agents in Ross, 1962, in Gen. Refs.). All kinds of mutations have been induced in organisms as different as phages, *Drosophila*, and mammals. The genetic risks of these mutagenic substances will be described at several places in this book.

Some bromides and chlorides are related to alkylating agents; for example, chloromethane, bromoethane, dichloro- and dibromoethane. Dibromoethane is widely used as a soil and grain fumigant; also dibromo- and dichloroethane

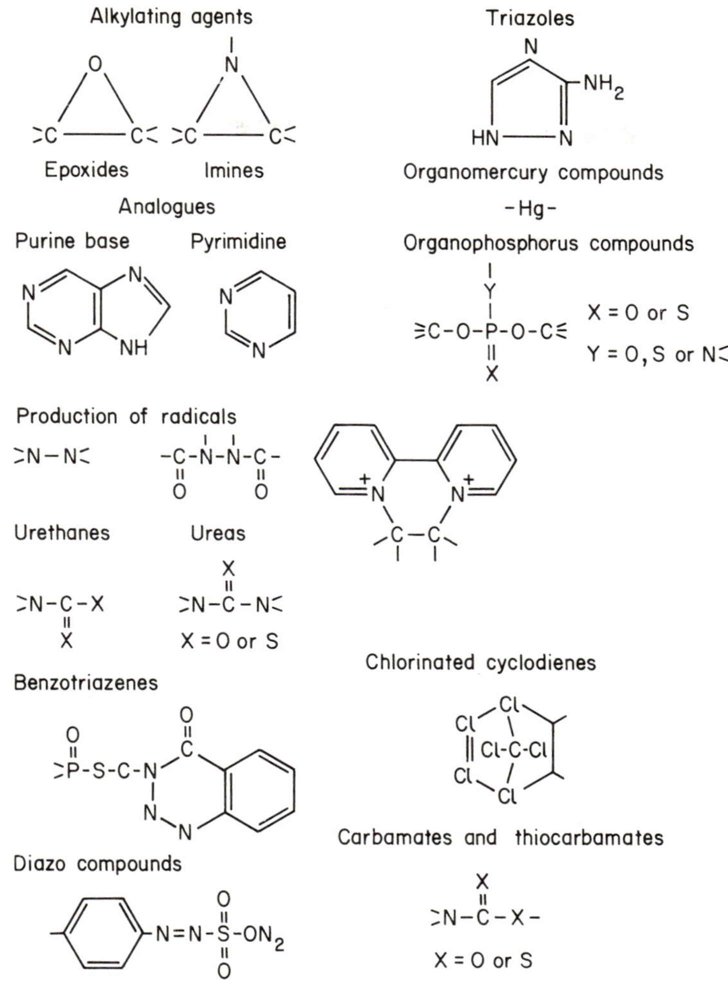

FIG 20. Principal active radicals of pesticides

can equally be classified in the group of substances used in industry as lead scavengers. Moreover, dichloroethane produces vinyl chloride, another major genetic hazard. The genotoxic effects of these substances have been investigated in several test systems (review in Rannug, 1980).

(2) Base analogues of purines and pyrimidines

Among the numerous analogues, fluorouracil and fluoroacetic acid are components of several pesticides.

(3) *Agents producing active radicals*

Hydrazines (review in Kimball, 1977) and maleic hydrazide (review in Swietlińska and Žuk, 1977), a well-known herbicide, should be mentioned first. They are known to induce gross chromosomal damage, but no point mutations have been detected so far. The genetic consequences are uncertain since major chromosomal aberrations can be selected out by cell death. γ–γ' dipyridyl salts such as paraquat, diquat and related substances can be included in this group.

(4) *Mercurials*

The mutagenicity and genetic hazards of these compounds will be described in Chapter 8.

(5) *Aromatic unsaturated rings with hydroxyl and thiol groups*

Chromosomal aberrations due to phenols have been described, but there is still little information about the mutation spectrum of these substances.

(6) *Urea derivatives*

Their effects at the chromosome level have not been so well investigated. As in the preceding section, their hydroxylation could activate them into products potentially capable of reacting with DNA.

(7) *Intercalating agents*

Acridine derivatives react with DNA, in which they intercalate between two adjacent bases. This may have various important genetic consequences. It seems that some anthraquinone derivatives, particularly pesticide components, are potential intercalating agents reacting with DNA as acridine derivatives.

Chlorinated dibenzo-*p*-dioxins belong to a class of compounds structuraliy related to acridines. From this structural analogy it was inferred that they might act as intercalating agents. They are formed during the manufacture of several commercial compounds such as herbicides, fungicides and germicides. They can also be found as impurities in some pestacides, e.g. 2,4,5-trichlorophenoxyacetic acid. They have sometimes been used for tree defoliation, resulting in environmental contamination. Their extreme toxicity has been known for a long time, but the tragic incident in Sevaso (Italy) in 1977 stimulated research into their potential mutagenicity, carcinogenicity and teratogenicity (review in Wassom *et al.*, 1977–78). They should also be classified in group II since they are used in industry. Only a small proportion of molecules of this class have been carefully analysed for mutagenicity, and the results are still controversial.

Another important question arises from the discovery that such substances are potent stimulant of hepatic enzymes such as aryl hydrocarbon hydroxylase (Poland and Glover, 1974). Such enzyme induction can activate a promutagen of a completely remote class into a mutagen. Epidemiological studies of occupational hazards have been undertaken, and should be continued since the results are still inconclusive.

(8) Arsenates and related compounds

Some of these compounds are known as inhibitors of certain enzymatic systems or as phosphorylating agents. Their genetic effects should be further investigated (see Chapter 8).

(9) Miscellaneous antibiotics

Some antibiotics may be added to pesticides, as in the case of griseofulvin.

The last three classes of pesticides are insecticides. Their mutagenicity has recently been surveyed (Moutschen, *et al.*, in Kirsch-Volders, 1984, in Gen. Refs.). To these three classes of powerful insecticides should be added some pyrethroid compounds, some of which have been tested for mutagenicity (Miyamoto, 1976). One of them, allethrin, showed strongly positive effects in Chinese hamster cells but only after activation with rat liver microsomal enzymes (Matsuoka *et al.*, 1979).

In lower organisms, 20% of the compounds showed positive mutagenic effects.

(10) Organophosphorus insecticides

Some of these rather labile compounds can react with DNA. Preferential attack of the phosphorus atom leads to phosphorylation, whereas preferential attack of the carbon atom leads to alkylation (reviews in Wild, 1975, and Moutschen *et al.*, in Kirsch-Volders, 1984). These classical properties are important in explaining the short persistence of organophosphorus insecticides in the environment. They differ from organochlorine compounds because they are rapidly biodegraded and cause fewer problems; for example, for the organophosphorus insecticide dichlorvos, the half-life was reported to be 13.5 min in rat kidney (Blair *et al.*, 1975). Some structure-activity relationships of several organophosphorus insecticides among those most widespread on the market could be demonstrated in the yeast, *Schizosaccharomyces pombe* (Gilot-Delhalle *et al.*, 1983). Results in mammals are much less clear, but it seems that detoxification processes are efficient. Organophosphorus compounds also produced positive genotoxic effects in *Drosophila*, which is certainly not the ideal test system for such compounds. Part of the biological effect of such compounds is certaily due to the alkylation processes, but the role of phosphorylation in genotoxicity is much less clear. In general, there is a good correlation between chemical and biological data, but differences of response are found between test systems, possibly due to different metabolization. As mentioned under pharmaceuticals, trichlorfon has particular hazards since it is used as an antischistosomal drug at doses higher than those when it is used as an insecticide.

(11) Carbamates and thiocarbamates

This is certainly an important group of susbtances. Among these compounds, carbaryl has been the most widely investigated. The majority of the experiments designed to show mutagenicity gave negative results. However, there is a possibility that this compound reacts with nitrosoderivatives to form nitrosocarbaryl. This compound was found to be highly mutagenic in *E. coli* (Elespuru *et al.*, 1974). It seems that such kinds of substance are rapidly detoxified in mammals (Degraeve *et al.*, 1976). The conditions under which mutagenicity can occur are not yet well known.

(12) Chlorinated insecticides

This group of compounds can be subdivided into several classes with various risks. First, DDT and related substances should be mentioned. Second, are chlorinated cyclodienes, among which are aldrin and endrin which can be transformed into epoxides in the body fat. There are also heptachlor and chlordane. All these compounds remain rather a long time in the body in which they modify some enzyme reactions (Chapter 8). It should be kept in mind that commercial insecticides are generally mixtures of different substances with potential synergistic effects.

Additives

Food additives

Substances added to food for various purposes (e.g. flavourings, emulsifyers, antimicrobials,) are innumerable. These additives are incorporated into very complex media in which numerous interactions occur. After absorption from the digestive tract, they can reach the gonads and there react possibly in a direct and acute way. They are not chance but permanent contaminations of the environment. Moreover, some additives which are neither toxic nor mutagenic become effective either after reaction with other ingredients or after absorption from the digestive tract (Chapters 7 and 8).

In the long series of food additives, five classes of substances should be especially mentioned: nitrites, cyclamates, saccharin, sequestrants (chelating agents), and nitrofurans.

A sixth class of substances has more recently been investigated. This comprises toxic substances that are formed in food, depending on the mode of preparation, e.g. cooking. Properly speaking, they are not food additives but can be classified in the same category with the same hazards. In 1977, Sugimura *et al.* identified highly mutagenic pyrolytic products in broiled foods. The same group of workers (Nagao *et al.*, 1977) demonstrated mutagenic properties of smoke condensates in fish and meat, and the occurrence of mutagens was confirmed in hamburgers (Commoner *et al.*, 1978). Six active molecules have been identified so far (two animo-dipyridoimidazole derivatives, Glu-P_1 and Glu-P_2, two amino-γ-carbolines, TrP–1 and TrP–2, and two amino-α-carbolines), and the identified compounds are expected to be formed in pyrolysates. All these substances clearly showed mutagenic activity in an Ames test with *Salmonella typhimurium* (TA 98), but the experiments have not yet been extended to higher organisms in which they are far more difficult to perform. All these findings raise important questions. Since man has been eating this kind of food for many generations, it is to be expected that his enzymatic equipment is adequate for inactivating the mutagens sufficiently quickly. Moreover, the uptake of such mutagens is low. Interactions with other food constituents still remain possible, however.

All these results stress once more the necessity of performing good metabolic studies in mammals to guide experiments in genetic toxicology.

(1) Nitrites

These derivatives are so important in the environment that their genetic effects will be described in more detail in a section of chapter 7.

(2) Cyclamates

These include cyclohexylamine and hydroxycyclohexylamine. Two of their metabolites in mammals are widely utilized as their calcium or sodium salts, either alone or combined with saccharin as a non-caloric substitute for sugar, especially in soft drinks. The clastogenic effects of these molecules were demonstrated in human cells, but the genetic consequences are still unknown (Table 3). However, in a review of cyclamates and their metabolites, Cattanach (1976) considered that the already numerous tests performed do not indicate a real mutagenic effect.

(3) Saccharin

This is used as an artificial sweetener and has been tested for mutagenicity in a variety of systems, which yielded sometimes controversial results possibly due to the presence of various impurities. It cannot be considered a proven mutagen, however (review in Kramers, 1975).

(4) Sequestrants.

Among these substances Versene (trisodium EDTA) is commonly found as an

TABLE 3. Investigations on some food additives

Substance	Organisms	Criteria	Authors
ETDA (versene)	Rat	Chromosomal aberrations	Tsarapin, 1967
	Tradescantia paludosa pollen cells	Chromosomal aberrations	Delone, 1958, 1959
	Onion root tips	Mitotic damage	McDonald and Kaufmann, 1957
	Drosophila	Chromosomal mutations	Kaufmann and McDonald, 1957; Khristol, 1961
	Vicia faba and barley seeds	Morphological and biochemical mutants	Wakonig and Arnason, 1958
Cyclohexylamine	Rodents (*in vitro* cells)	Chromosomal aberrations	Legator, 1968
	Rat (*in vivo* spermatogonia)	Chromosomal aberrations	Legator *et al.*, 1969
Cyclamates	Onion root tips	Chromosomal aberrations	Sax and Sax, 1968
	Human cells *in vitro*	Chromosomal aberrations	Stone *et al.*, 1969

additive in a large variety of foods (e.g. numerous tinned foods, dressings, mayonnaise, spices) as well as in e.g. pharmaceuticals, pesticides. As with cyclamates, its clastogenicity has been well established in several biological systems (Table 3). We demonstrated (Moutschen *et al.*, 1969) that some chelating agents can interfere with mutagenic agents, particularly ionizing radiations. The consequences of lesions possibly produced by chelating agents are not well known, but it is not excluded that they could play a role in mutagenesis.

(5) Nitrofurans

Some nitrofuran derivatives, among which are nitrofurazone, nitrofurylacrylamide and furylfuramide, have been used as food additives in some countries particularly in Japan (review in Tazima *et al.*, 1975). The mutagenic potential of nitrofuran derivatives is described in Chapter 5. Their use as food additives underlines the need for rigorous control of foods for potential mutagenicity.

Other, non-alimentary additives

It should be kept in mind that potentially mutagenic substances may be added to pharmaceuticals and even to some pesticides. Such kinds of additives are in many respects comparable to those sporadically appearing in the environment, and are thereby classified in group II. Some of them might be a potential hazard especially due to possible interactions and synergistic effects.

Cosmetics belong to various chemical classes of compounds which have been investigated by different groups of researchers over the last decades. Hair dyes, especially those containing aromatic amines, have been known for a long time to induce urinary bladder cancer, but relevant epidemiological studies only started more recently (review in Clemmesen, 1981). Epidemiological investigation was sponsored by the International Commission for Protection against Environmental Mutagens and Carcinogens. In human populations, cosmetics can act at two distinct levels: first as an occupational hazard to workers in factories producing such substances, and second, to persons who apply cosmetics to themselves or to customers of barber shops.

The genotoxicity of cosmetic colouring agents has recently been reviewed (Combes and Haveland-Smith, 1982). There is an interesting observation concerning the strategy that should be used in mutagenicity testing. A hair dye, 2–(2′, 4′-diaminophenoxy)ethanol, was devoid of mutagenic activity in various test systems, whereas a related compound the 2,4-diaminoanisolemethoxy derivative, taken as a positive control, showed mutagenicity (Loprieno *et al.*, 1982). This is an example where the conclusion is clearly drawn from mutagenicity testing that one compound should be preferred and the other rejected.

Biological contaminants

In 1961, Hampar and Elisson described chromosomal lesions due to *Herpes simplex* virus. Since these observations, multiple chromosomal lesions have been described in more than 40 virus infections not only in man but also in birds and mice. There exist excellent reviews about this subject: Nichols, 1963; Makino and Aya, 1968; Moorhead, 1970, in Gen. Refs.; Stich and John, 1970; Bartsch in Vogel and Röhrborn, 1970; Nichols, 1982.

The cytological effects observed are of at least seven types.

(1) First, there are localized effects such as those described in Chapter 2. These effects very much resemble those induced by classical mutagenic agents. One cannot state, however, that the mechanism which produces such lesions is the same in both cases (Fig 21a).
(2) One finds also diffuse cellular lesions. Chromosomes are completely pulverized so that mitotic stages are no longer recognizable (Fig. 21b). This latter effect is not only observed in virus diseases but also in rickettsiosis (Halkka, 1967) and mycoplasmosis (Fogh and Fogh, 1967). It is probably an effect of the lytic type.
(3) There are colchicomitotic effects which can generate cells with a modified number of chromosomes, i.e. heteroploid cells. Most of these effects are commonly observed in well-known diseases. Thus, in measles, Nichols (1963) observed clastogenicity induced by the virus, whereas in patients vaccinated and treated by γ-globulins the level of damage was not significantly higher than in healthy persons.
(4) There is also a strange effect called premature chromosome condensation first described in tissue cells cultured free from all biological contamination. It is considered to be an indirect viral effect resulting from cell fusion between two cells at different stages of the mitotic cycle. The mitotic cell synthesizes a protein which induces an interphase nucleus entering mitosis. The mechanism by which the virus acts is not well understood.
(5) During the malignant transformation of cultured cells infected by Rauscher leukemia virus (Brown and Crossen, 1976) or simian virus (SV40) (Wolff *et al.* 1977; Nichols *et al.*, 1978), an increased frequency of sister-chromatid exchanges has been described.
(6) There is increasing evidence that, as well as clastogenic effects, some viruses can also induce point mutations (quoted in Nichols, 1982), even though this possibility was contested some years ago.
(7) Finally, there is also the possibility of gene transfer from virus to the host cell. In some infections it has been demonstrated that viral DNA or DNA copies of viral RNA can be covalently inserted into the DNA of the host nucleus; for example, the gene that codes for thymidine kinase in the *Herpes simplex* virus has been found to be integrated into mammalian cell DNA (Bacchetti and Graham, 1977, 1978).

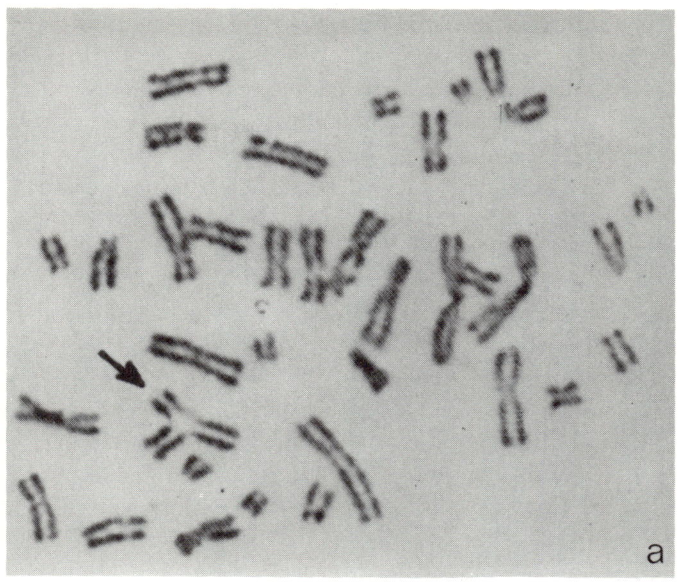

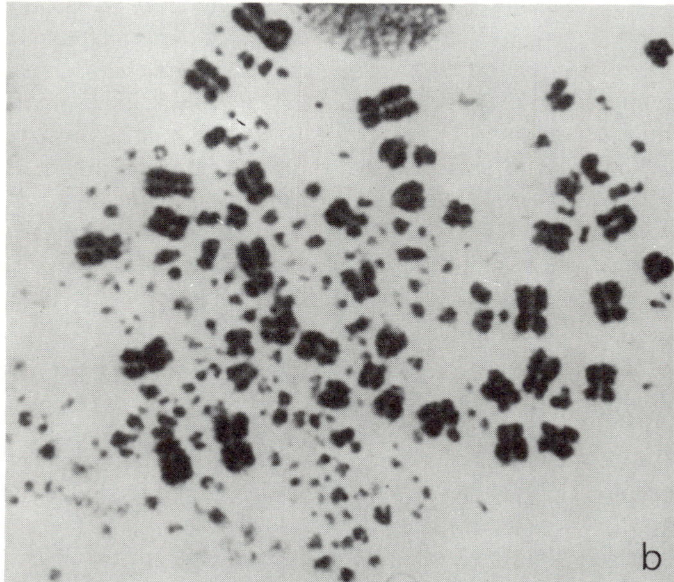

FIG. 21. Chromosome damage due to biological contaminants.
a. Chromosomal aberration (chromatid interchange indicated by the arrow) observed in a leucocyte of a patient suffering from measles.
b. Chromosome breakage observed after experimental infection of cultured human leucocytes by measles virus. In a syncytium resulting from the fusion of two cells, a group of chromosomes shows more breakage than the other. Chromosomes of picture b should be compared with chromosomes of picture a. (Pictures by courtesy of Dr. W. Nichols, Department of Cytogenetics, Institute of Medical Research, Camden, NJ, USA, with the permission of *Hereditas*.) (× 1700)

A large proportion of research on cytogenetic effects of viruses has been performed using experimentally infected cultured cells. Furthermore, major chromosomal lesions have also been observed in blood or bone marrow cells of patients suffering from measles (Nichols, 1963), yellow fever (Harnden, 1964), viral hepatitis (El-Alfi *et al.*, 1965; Matsaniotis *et al.*, 1966; Mella and Lang, 1967) and smallpox (Zur Hausen and Lanz, 1966). These lesions sometimes remain for a long time after the cessation of the symptoms of these diseases.

It must be noted that the clastogenic activity is as high for RNA viruses (as in measles or yellow fever) as for DNA viruses (as in smallpox or herpes). Leukaemogenic and tumorigenic viruses should be mentioned separately. Marek's virus, responsible for chicken leukosis, induces chromosomal aberrations in the carrier animal (Owen *et al.*, 1966). At least five types of Rous sarcoma virus have been tested for clastogenicity (review in Bartsch, 1970). Whereas Kato (1967, 1968) observed chromosome breaks specifically localized in Chinese hamster cells, Lithmer and Pontén (1966) did not notice specific alterations in lung fibroblasts from ox infected by this virus. This indicates a great variation of response.

It is often admitted that important genetic modifications induced by leukaemogenic and tumorigenic viruses are equivalent *in vitro* to a malignant transformation (review in Nichols, 1982). Could it not happen that clastogenic viruses released from mammalian tissue cultures adapt themselves to human cells producing important genetic changes eventually leading to disasters? In the same context, it should be remembered that man had already dispersed insect viruses in nature for insecticidal purposes (Ignoffo, 1968).

As can be seen, the problem of biological contaminants is far beyond the scope of genetics alone. It is a complex problem which is fast growing into a new branch of science and has multiple approaches. Some of the above-mentioned results could lead to some aspects of anti-infection prophylaxis, being reconsidered.

GROUP II: MUTAGENS USED IN INDUSTRY OR OCCURRING AS BY-PRODUCTS OF INDUSTRY

Genetic risks of substances classified in this group arise at two levels: first, in the industries themselves where they are produced, and second in the environment among the substances released by industries.

In the jungle of pollutants released by industries a special place should be reserved for aldehydes and dialdehydes, on the one hand, and epoxides, peroxides and hydroperoxides on the other. Among the aldehydes, ordinary formaldehyde has been amply investigated. Historically its effects were first described in *Drosophila* by Rapoport (1946), Kaplan (1948) and Auerbach (1949, 1952). These mutagenic effects have since been widely confirmed (review in Auerbach *et al.*, 1977). It is not yet known if formaldehyde acts as an alkylating agent or in a quite different way, but its spectrum of mutation is broad. It is also widespread in various industrial processes: synthetic resins, textiles, papers, synthesis of a great number of components.

The mutagenicity of acetaldehyde, acrolein and some ketones is less clear. Cytological effects of two aldehydes — butyraldehyde and crotonaldehyde which can also be produced in various conditions by irradiation of sugars with ionizing radiations — have been observed (Moutschen *et al.*, 1975, 1976). Among other things in mice, they were able to induce polyploid cells by a mechanism which has not yet been elucidated. It could be due to cell or even nuclear fusion or by inhibition of cell wall formation. If it is demonstrated by further research that this property is common to various molecules, a new cytogenetic problem will be raised which might be of considerable importance.

Among substances of the second type, hydrogen peroxide is one of the simplest. It is known to be responsible for some of the effects of ionizing radiations (review in Bacq and Alexander, 1955 in Gen. Refs.). It is used as a germicide in the sterilization of e.g. starch, flour, as a bleaching agent (e.g. for hairs), in the plastics industry. For various reasons it is found in many places in our daily environment. The series of organic peroxides and hydroperoxides in the polymer industry (e.g. plastics, rubber, synthetic resins), is growing longer and longer. As examples of compounds for which the mutation spectrum has been analysed, can be mentioned succinic acid peroxide, ter-butyl hydroperoxide and cumene hydroperoxide.

Among the epoxides, ethylene oxide has certainly been responsible for much damage, the outcome of which is often tragic since we are dealing here with an extremely volatile alkylating agent. In a Swedish factory making ethylene glycol, the blood of workers was analysed at regular intervals for many years. The haematological analyses revealed anomalies, and an increase in the frequency of leukaemia was expected (Ehrenberg and Hällström cited by Kallins in *Radiosterilization of Medical Products*, 1967). Certainly in this and similar cases, haematological monitoring of workers could help prevent such leukemias to some extent. Ehrenberg's group (1967, 1974, 1981) showed that workers exposed to ethylene oxide can accumulate a weekly dose of 5 rad-equivalents (definition in Chapter 10). A comparable control of workers exposed to vinyl chloride was also performed in Swedish factories (Funès-Cravioto *et al.*, 1975).

It has been demonstrated that after chronic exposure to a mutagenic agent, chromosomal aberrations continue to appear for relatively long periods of time. According to Ehrenberg and Hällström (1967), prolonged exposure to ethylene oxide produces effects comparable to 50–100 rad of whole body irradiation by γ-rays. Ethylene oxide, propylene oxide, and various substances of this class are certainly among the most genetically active pollutants widespread in the environment. They are typical of substances that represent a risk not only for industrial workers but also in the environment as a whole, due to the industrial by-products. The importance of such substances in industry is great for they are used in the syntheses of such compounds as ethylene glycol, diethylene glycol, methylcarbitol, dioxane, ethylene chlorhydrin, carbowax, acrylonitrile and monoethylamine. They are also utilized in the synthesis of cellulosic materials, in the textile industry and in plastic solvents where they remain for long periods of time. Kulkarni *et al.* (1968) showed that even after sterilization they can be easily detected after a week. This kind of risk concerns only that part of the population in direct contact with these substances but which from the viewpoint of population genetics is already considerable.

But these substances are also utilized to sterilize pharmaceuticals and even foods, due to their antimicrobial properties. This means that a large proportion of the population may be exposed (*Radiosterilization of Medical Products*, 1967). In food, toxic chlorhydrins remain a long time after treatment (Wesley *et al*, 1965; Ragelis *et al.*, 1968). In some cases, diepoxides such as 2,3-epoxypropyl ether and 1,2:3,4-diepoxybutane even have some industrial applications, the first in photography and the polymer industry as floculating agents and in the synthesis of organic substances, the second as preservative, against microbial proliferation, and in the textile and polymer industries. It should also be remembered that epoxides sometimes occur as atmospheric pollutants. The series of homologous epoxide derivatives is grouped in the next chapter. Among the industrial substances identified as mutagens we should mention hydrazine and its derivatives (used in photography, textiles, combustibles, explosives, plastics). According to Freese *et al.* (1968), this kind of substance can produce hydrogen peroxide by interaction with oxygen. This mechanism would explain DNA inactivation of pneumococcal transforming factors. Hydroxylamine, which is used for numerous chemical syntheses, in the nylon industry, photography, should also be mentioned (review in Marfey and Robinson, 1981). Finally, it should be kept in mind that some metal salts are frequently found in the environment as industrial by-products (see Chapter 8).

GROUP III: NATURALLY OCCURRING MUTAGENS

Alkaloids and related substances

In comparison to the genetic risks of substances which one way or another are the consequence of the expanding human technology, potential mutagenic substances which have always existed in the environment seem less risky. It is well known that a large part of the plant kingdom contains alkaloids. Some plant families have a special tendency for supplying man with a multiplicity of beneficial, or harmful, substances.

A typical substance which has generated many articles is surely caffeine, together with related alkaloids like theophylline and theobromine. In order to express an objective opinion, it is not without interest to summarize the story of this substance in mutagenesis. In 1948, Fries and Kihlman detected mutagenic effects of caffeine in the fungus *Ophiostoma multiannulatum*. Almost at the same time clastogenic properties were described in onion root tips by Kihlman and Levan (1949). Independently, the experiments of Demerec and his coworkers (1948, 1951) showed mutagenicity in *E. coli*. A comparative study of clastogenic effects of purine derivatives (Kihlman, 1952) aroused the interest of geneticists who attempted to evaluate carefully the potential hazards of these compounds. For technical reasons there was at that time no possibility of performing conclusive experiments in mammals. Results obtained with lower organisms and plants had to be extrapolated to man. In animals, further research yielded contradictory conclusions. According to Andrew (1959) and Clark and Clark (1968), caffeine induces chromosomal aberrations in *Drosophila* but no mutation is inherited. In cultured human cells, chromosome lesions were observed by Ostertag and coworkers (1965, 1966), but, in mouse, mutagenicity was still spurious (Lyon *et al.*, 1962; Cattanach, 1962; review by Adler, 1970; Epstein, 1970; Timson, 1977).

The 8-ethoxy derivative of caffeine, for its part, raised a particular problem in mutagenesis. Synthesized by Kihlman, this substance induced chromosome damage (Kihlman, 1955; Moutschen and Moutschen-Dahmen, 1958). On the one hand, it was shown that chromosomal lesions due to this compound are very localized, probably due to specific reactions at the molecular level. On the other hand, Ehrenberg *et al.* (1956) found that the mutation rate due to this highly clastogenic substance is quite low in plants. We are therefore faced with a particular situation since it seems that most of the effects at the chromosome level are eliminated at the treated generation and are not transmitted to the next.

The metabolism of caffeine and related compounds has been investigated in detail in mammals, including man. Fifteen per cent of the dose is excreted every hour, and its distribution in different tissues is well known. Its detoxification is rapid, whereas reactions leading to mutations are generally slower. The many controversies concerning the nature of the mutagenic effects of caffeine derivatives justified a whole session of the 3rd European Environmental Mutagen Society meeting held in Uppsala, 1973) aimed at surveying this question. It appears that caffeine is mutagenic only in specific organisms, precisely those that lack the powerful detoxification mechanisms. Apart from quite exceptional flooding of the detoxification mechanism as might occur in acute intoxications or in the case of specific enzyme inhibition by other substances taken at the same time, caffeine can not be considered really mutagenic in mammals and man. Nevertheless, two particular instances suggest caution from a genetic standpoint: (1) in cases where patients (e.g. persons suffering from heart diseases) are treated with high doses for a long period (e.g. by aminophylline); (2) in cases where these pharmaceuticals show synergistic effects with other agents (Chapter 8).

For other alkaloids, mutagenicity, though relatively low, has been demonstrated. Solanine which sometimes occurs in food, induced clastogenic effects on plant cells (unpublished data). It is not certain if these effects can be generalized and extrapolated to man. Additional data are required. The property of extracts of citrus peel, especially of mandarin oranges, to inhibit cell division at a specific stage, doubling the chromosome number (polyploidizing effect), has been known for a long time. This property was formerly exploited in plant technology to improve varieties. It could, in principle, be extended to all living animal or plant cells, unless significant differences in detoxification processes exist. In fact, this is precisely what seems to happen in man for colchicine, the 'leader' among polyploidizing agents, still used in the treatment of gout. In fact, for such substances, we have only to consider the exceptional human pathological cases where detoxification processes become ineffective for one reason or another.

Various alkaloids are still used in local medicine or are sometimes found in food as condiments. They could also be grouped with drugs. Cycasin (methylazoxymethanol glucoside) extracted from several *Cycas* species is certainly mutagenic in *Salmonella typhimurium* (Smith, 1966) and *Drosophila melanogaster* (Teas and Dyson, 1967). Its aglycone has powerful clastogenic effect in onions (Teas *et al.*, 1965). The effects of cycasin and its mutagenic metabolites have recently been reviewed (Morgan and Hoffmann, 1983). The mutagenicity of alkaloids of the pyrrolizidine group will be compared in the next chapter.

Another quite different mutagenic compound is allylisothiocyanate which occurs in foods such as cabbage, parsnips, mustard (and in general in the Cruciferaceae). It is also used as a food additive in various dressings. In fact, it is one of the first substances identified as mutagen and clastogen in *Drosophila* (Auerbach and Robson, 1944). It induced mutations in the fungus *Ophiostoma* (Fries, 1948) and produced chromosome aberrations in onion (Sharma and Sharma, 1962).

The mutagenic effects of steroid diamines such as malouetine, irehdiamine and other alkaloids from Apocynaceae is not yet irrefutably proved. On the other hand, extracts of ferns like *Pteridium aquilinum* and *Osmunda japonica*, show incontestable mutagenic effects in *Drosophila* and mouse (Evans, 1968), possibly due to an alkylating agent, the nature of which has not yet been elucidated.

In some countries, cattle suffer from a kind of 'radiomimetic' syndrome after eating bracken fern (*Pteridium aquilinum*). The condition is mainly characterized by gastrointestinal lesions and also by bone marrow depletion sometimes leading to death (Evans and Mason, 1965; Evans, 1968). The mutagenicity of bracken fern extracts is obvious in *Drosophila* and mouse. In the mouse, and perhaps also in quail, Evans (1968) observed an action on spermatogenesis, and induced dominant lethal mutations. The nature of the implicated factor(s) has not been elucidated; according to Van Duuren (quoted in Fishbein *et al.*, 1970, in Gen. Refs.) it is a precursor of an alkylating agent. Moreover, the discovery in this fern of two insect hormones, α-ecdysone I and 20-hydroecdysone II, was surprising since this kind of molecule has never been tested for mutagenicity (Kaplanis *et al.*, 1967).

An unexpected problem is the possible mutagenicity of natural products occurring in food though not being considered food additives. As an example, five natural food colours permitted within the European Economic Community, namely anthocyanin, Annatto, beetroot red, β-carotene and riboflavin, were investigated for mutagenicity in bacteria. Fortunately, no mutagenicity could be detected (Haveland-Smith, 1981). In fact, the question of mutagenicity of such naturally occurring substances has long been debated in the case of quercetin, a quite ubiquitous substance (review in Brown, 1980).

For many centuries we have been eating such compounds. Therefore it would be surprising to find them mutagenic in man! Should not we be adapted? But how far will we adapt to everything? After all, is not the rabbit able to digest perfectly one of the most terrible poisons that the plant kingdom gave to man: the toxins of the deadly agaric (*Amanita phalloides*)?

Products of bacterial metabolism

It should be remembered that some products of microbial (bacteria, fungi, yeasts) metabolism can fortuitously be found in foods. In Table 3 references are given on the effects of some antibiotics. We can also mention substsances that have no antibiotic properties such as nitrosamines, aflatoxins and some toxins more recently discovered in Roquefort cheese. The problems raised by such compounds, fortunately occurring only in rather rare but unpredicted circumstances, will be discussed in Chapter 7.

In conclusion, compared with the risks of the substances of the two first groups, the risk of natural substances is generally minor, and only occurs in specific circumstances which certainly should be better known, but which would not result in significant genetic effects for the whole population.

Chapter 5

Analogies and Homologies in the Field of Mutagenesis: Structure–Activity Relationships

Mutagenic substances occurring episodically or more permanently in the environment belong to the most varied chemical classes.

On the one hand, there are substances with quite different formulae which have comparable mutagenic effects, though the spectra of induced mutations are in general different. From the genetic viewpoint, this should be called an analogy. For instance, quite different alkylating agents derived from such unrelated nuclei as diepoxybutane and triethylene melamine are two well-known strong mutagenic and clastogenic compounds. When tested in the same organism, it is possible to find a concentration which yields the same mutagenic effects.

On the other hand, there are homologous series of compounds, all derived from the same nucleus, but differing in structural details such as radicals or functional groups located at different positions on the molecule. As a function of these structural differences, the molecules of an homologous series can also display great differences in mutagenic activity. In other words, in the same chemical class there are substances genetically inactive as well as substances inducing mainly point mutations, or, in contrast, a majority of chromosomal aberrations. In this respect, ethyl methanesulphonate and Myleran bis-(methanesulphonyloxy)butane, belong to the class of alkyl alkane sulphonates. The first induces point mutations at high frequencies whereas the second produces mutations which more frequently correspond to chromosome damage visible under the microscope. In the same class, 2,2-dimethylpropyl methanesulphonate does not induce mutagenic effects at all (Moutschen, 1965a) due to its low reactivity (Ehrenberg *et al.*, 1966; Osterman-Golkar *et al.*, 1970).

Knowledge of the reactive groups and of their position in the molecule should in principle allow the mutagenic properties of a substance to be predicted. By comparison with functional molecules in biochemistry, one could define homologues as substances which induce different genetic effects at least quantitatively though having the same basic structure.

Knowledge of homologous series should in general help in assessing the genetic risks involved. In the past, studies of the relationships between structure and activity in the field of pharmacology were rewarding, e.g. for antibiotics. The following examples will not provide an exhaustive review of the matter since the effects of some chemical groups are still so badly known or

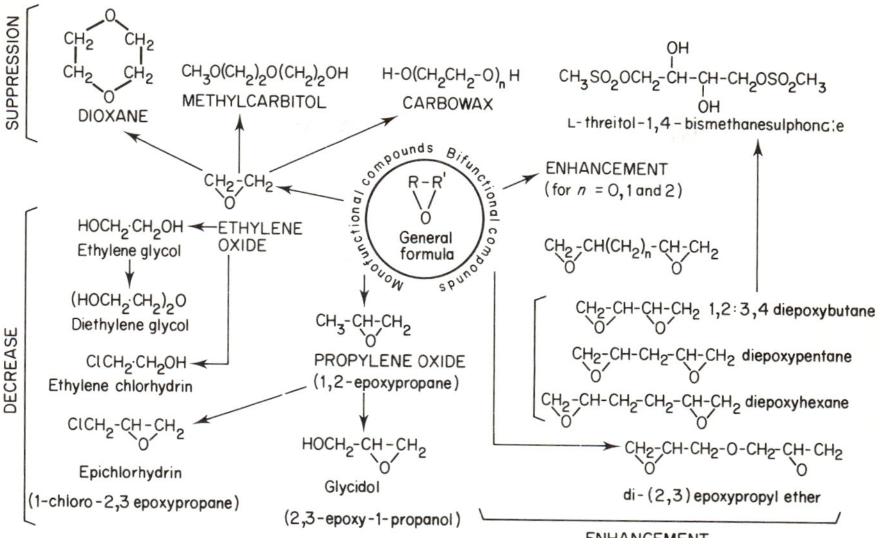

FIG. 22. Modifications in mutagenic properties of the epoxide series related to molecular modifications

ill-defined that whole classes of mutagenic agents remain unexplored. We have selected a few chemical classes for which we are going to attempt to correlate the structure of the molecules with the multiple mutagenic effects and see what alterations in the chemical structure modify these genetic effects.

Epoxides

Among alkylating agents, the class of epoxides is of special interest for environmental mutagenesis (Chapter 4). Transformation of the epoxide group into hydroxyl decreases the activity (Fig. 22) with the exception of a diol, threitol 1,4-dimethanesulphonate, fortunately not risky for man. This diol can be transformed, especially in tissues, into the bis-epoxide. In specific circumstances, it shows drastic delayed effects on chromosomes. These effects could be adequately exploited for fundamental investigations into chromosome breakage (Moutschen and Reekmans, 1964; Moutschen, 1965b), and for plant breeding. This compound was also utilized in cancer research (Feit, 1960, 1961, 1964). Halogen derivatives of epoxides retain the major mutagenic activity as in the cases of chlorhydrin and epichlorhydrin. A series of substances derived from epoxides and commonly used in industry and in laboratories is fortunately without mutagenic activity (dioxane*, methylcarbitol, carbowax). Bifunctional derivatives show higher toxicity and mutagenicity than monofunctional derivatives and also modifications of mutation spectra. This is only true when the two active groups are not separated by more than two carbon atoms.

* Genetic effects of dioxane were detected in barley (Ehrenberg *et al.*, 1956). They might be due to peroxides rapidly formed in solutions of this substance or to some other impurities.

The clastogenic activity of diepoxybutane is distinctly higher than the activity of either ethylene oxide or propylene oxide, but is comparable with the activity of an ether, diepoxypropyl ether. Such correlations between structure and mutagenic effects should be established for each class of alkylating agents, if possible comparatively in various test systems.

For the series of sulphonates, in plants and partly in mammals, modifications of the mutagenic activity are well correlated with specific modifications of the molecular structures (Moutschen, 1965a). Although, for the majority of alkylating agents, mutagenicity is associated with carcinogenicity, this is curiously not the case in this class of molecules which are highly mutagenic but weakly, if not at all, carcinogenic.

Acridines

The class of acridines is another example of an homologous series. Clastogenic properties of these molecules were first described by D'Amato (1950) in his pioneer work. They were further compared using the same test system (D'Amato, 1951, 1952; D'Amato and Avanzi, 1954). Some general rules evolve from this and other research (Fig. 23). Acridine itself is highly clastogenic, as are proflavine and acridine orange, although results were not always reproducible. The replacement of a methyl group by a chloro group decreases the activity as in trypaflavine. A series of 9-amino derivatives, chlorinated at various positions, show fewer effects than the three substances mentioned above. On the other hand, it seems well established that derivatives containing a 9-amino group at the same time as a methoxy group at positions 2, 3 or 4 show enhanced activity. Comparison is made difficult since, in the experiments reported here, these substances were tested at a much lower concentration. The introduction of a methoxy group at position 2 and a chloro group at position 6 results in a loss of clastogenic activity.

The transformation of acridine into acridine mustard considerably enhances the clastogenic properties. It is not surprising since the group —CH_2—CH_2—Cl confers on the molecule a strong alkylating property, giving the molecule a double polarity. Various acridine mustards have been synthesized and the above rule remains valid. Fortunately, all these dangerous substances are only used in laboratories. Nevertheless, they raise the problem of the protection of the technicians who too often do not take the elementary precautions prescribed by the health authorities because they believe that the 'chemical monsters are tamed'. Unfortunately, this remark is true in too many instances. The laboratory is especially the melting-pot in which interactions between mutagenic agents can happen. In this context, one should insist on the necessity for researchers who are routinely manipulating duly identified mutagenic agents to adhere strictly to the protection rules. This is certainly the case for alkylating agents and ionizing radiations of any kind (e.g. radioisotopes).

The transformation of acridine into quinacrine diminishes the mutagenicity but does not suppress it completely. This is fortunate since quinacrine hydroch-

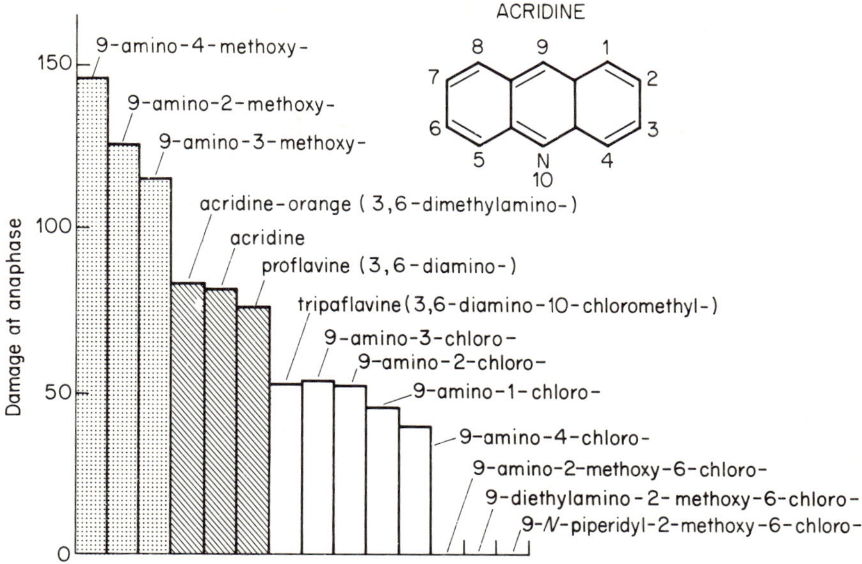

FIG. 23. Variations in clastogenic activity (on onion root-tip cells observed at anaphase) of some acridine derivatives related to the position of active groups. Onion root tips are treated at a concetration 10 mg/l except for the three last compounds (black areas) for which data are extrapolated from results obtained at a concentration 1 mg/l. (After D'Amato, 1950, 1952; D'Amato and Avanzi, 1954.)

loride (Atabrine, Acranil, Mepacrine) is widely used for malaria therapy, sometimes at high doses and for long periods. The mutagenic activity reappears after introduction of an alkylating group as in quinacrine mustard and related molecules.

In higher plants, Kihlman (1959) showed that light plus oxygen are required with acridine orange to produce chromosomal aberrations. These results have been confirmed by Nuti-Ronchi and D'Amato (1961), but these factors were not taken into account in previous experiments of D'Amato. According to Kihlman (1959), light of specific wavelength is strongly absorbed by the dye, then secondarily transferred to DNA in which excited molecular states and free radicals can be produced. These transfers of energy lead either to chromosomal aberrations or point mutations. Rapid progress in the techniques of fluorescence and electron spin resonance have helped in our understanding of the relationship between the chemical structure and mutagenicity of acridines.

As well as research on the clastogenic effects of acridine derivatives in plants, many experiments have been designed to detect their mutagenic effects in micro-organisms. Mutagenic effects of proflavine have been described in phage T2 and in cultured human cells (De Mars, 1953; Ostertag and Kersten, 1965). Mutagenicity of acriflavine was found in *E. coli* (Witkin, 1947; Demerec *et al.*, 1951), in yeast (Avers and Dryfuss, 1965) and in *Drosophila* (Witkin *et al.*, 1947). In all these works, photosensitization was not taken much into account.

In a search for new antitumour drugs, 9-aminoalkyl acridines and derivatives were prepared and tested for mutagenicity in *Salmonella typhimurium* (Kalinowska and Chorazy, 1980). 9-[3['-(dimethyl-aminopropylamine)propyl] amino]acridine was a weak mutagen in this test system, but the addition of a nitro group in position 1 or 2 considerably enhanced the mutagenic activity although the 2-nitro derivative is much less mutagenic than the 1-nitro derivative. This seems to be related to differences in DNA repair processes. According to these researchers, it proves that the nitro group is involved in the interaction with the bacterial genome. There is also a correlation between the mutagenicity and the cytostatic properties, which offers some possibilities in tumour therapeutics.

Calberg-Bacq *et al.* (1968) showed that the efficiency of various acridines in photoinactivation of T4B phage can be classified in order of increasing activity: acridine red $<$ 9-amino-acridine $<$ acridine yellow $\ll$ acriflavine $<$ acridine orange. The photoinactivation efficiency is correlated with the intensity of the signal of electron spin resonance. However, in these experimental conditions, the mutagenic activity of acridines is found to be of the same order of magnitude, except for 9-aminoacridine which is much less efficient.

In the wide class of acridines, it is possible that mutagenic and clastogenic effects are produced by different mechanisms. A correlation still seems difficult to ascertain.

It is of interest to remember that in phage, at least, the mechanism which produces mutations is peculiar. By insertion between two nucleotides, acridines can, among other things, produce frameshift mutations. This kind of mutation has not been demonstrated in higher organisms, particularly mammals, in which they may result in unexpected consequences.

In more recent experiments, proflavine showed unusual properties as mutagenic agent in some strains of *Salmonella typhimurium*. It was found to induce direct frameshift mutations in the presence of microsomal enzymes without photosensitization (Speck and Rosenkranz, 1980). Visible light changes the spectrum of mutations, however. The results of this research were taken to indicate that proflavine possesses direct frameshift activity by intercalating between DNA bases, but only after metabolic activation. If this possibility is extended to other acridines and other test systems, especially *in vivo*, the problem of the relationship between structure and activity should be kept in mind owing to the wide use of such molecules (e.g. in herpetic infection, as a topical antiseptic agent especially in newborn infants).

Pyrrolizidines

These alkaloids are the third example of homologous series. They are produced by plants of various families — Compositae, Boraginaceae, Leguminosae (especially in the genus *Crotalaria*) — and more recently have been found in others — Gramineae, Celastraceae, Orchideae, Rhizophoraceae, Sapotaceae and Santalaceae. They are still used in popular medicine in some countries, for instance in Australia. Some of these substances are thought to be responsible for liver troubles observed in herbivores (Bull, 1955; *et al.*, 1956). Their hepatotoxic effects in man are well known according to the results of Schoental and Head (1955) and Schoental and Magee (1957). Some of them (heliotrine and monocrotaline) are clastogenic in plants (Avanzi, 1962) and in kangaroo-rat cultured cells (Bick and Jackson, 1968; Bick and Brown, 1972). A comparative study of mutagenic effects of some pyrrolizidines in *Drosophila* has been made by Clark (1960). He measured the frequency of sex-linked recessive lethal mutations. Only compounds which have a hidden esterified allyl group can act as alkylating agents, being thereby hepatotoxic and mutagenic at the same time. In Fig. 24, an analysis of sex-linked lethal mutations is given for two hatching periods. It can be seen that, on the basis of these data, the group of alkaloids can be divided into three subgroups of strong, medium and low mutagenic activity, respectively. According to Culvenor *et al.* (1962), the mutagenic activity generally correlated with hepatotoxicity depends upon the lateral chains of the molecules, resulting more particularly in modifications of

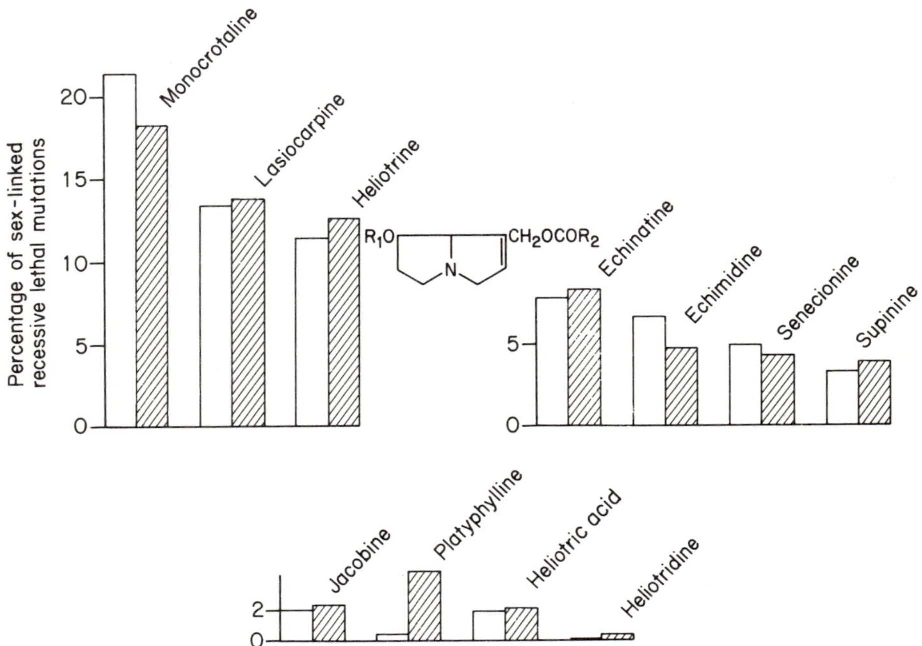

FIG. 24. Relationships between molecular structure and mutagenic activity of pyrrolizidine alkaloids in *Drosophila*. White and hatched areas: percentages of mutations observed in a Muller-5 test for two successive hatchings after treatment of males. Pyrrolizidines differ by the two radicals R_1 and R_2 (see text)

hydrosolubility. McKenzie (1958) investigated in detail the pharmacological properties of these substances and showed that their anticholinergic activity requires the integrity of the ester moiety. Therefore, the pharmacological and mutagenic properties are independent of each other, as shown in Table 4. In this table, the values given are compared with lasiocarpine taken as unity in both cases. For pharmacological activity, the data are from McKenzie (1958), and for mutagenic activity from Clark (1960). Both show an evident inverse relationship. For example, platyphylline shows an anticholinergic activity 1000 times higher than lasiocarpine along with a mutagenic activity 14 times lower.

Fig. 24 attempts to correlate the mutagenic efficiency of some pyrrolizidine alkaloids with their molecular structure. In the series of alkaloids investigated by Culvenor *et al.* (1962) it appears with a few exceptions that the structure required for hepatotoxicity is given in Fig. 24 where radical R^1 is a branched allyl chain and radical R_2 is H, OH or O-acyl with a double bond in the pyrrolizidine ring and an esterified hydroxy group branched with an acidic chain.

Thus, in the field of therapeutics, it should be easy to select molecules which at appropriate doses show maximal efficiency with minimal mutagenic risks.

Despite several investigations of Culvenor *et al.* (1962) with ^{14}C-labelled lasiocarpine, the metabolic details remain to be ascertained.

In this series of substances, a relationship was established between the antimitotic activity which explains the toxicity for mammal parenchyma and sex-linked recessive lethal mutations in *Drosophila*.

It is worth seeing if the conclusions drawn from *Drosophila* experiments and pharmacological studies can be extrapolated to mammals. The results are somewhat scanty to allow a general picture to emerge, but recent experiments have yielded important information.

The genotoxicity of four pyrrolizidine alkaloids — heliotrine, lasiocarpine, petasitenine and senkirkine — has been tested on V79 Chinese hamster cells

TABLE 4. Comparison of anticholinergic activity in rat and mutagenic activity in *Drosophila*. The activities are compared with lasiocarpine activity taken as unity in both cases. (Rat: data of McKenzie, 1958; *Drosophila*: data of Clark, 1960.)

Substance	Anticholinergic activity in rat	Mutagenic activity in *Drosophila*
Lasiocarpine	1.0	1.0
Heliotrine	3.0	0.9
Senecionine	3.4	0.4
Monocrotaline	0.07	1.6
Jacobine	0.3	0.08
Supinine	78	0.2
Heleurine	170	–
Platyphylline	1000	0.07
(Atropine)	5300	0.00

cultured *in vitro* for both clastogenicity and 8-azaguanine-resistant mutations. The four alkaloids induced both types of effects. These effects are induced independently from the addition of microsomal enzymes (Takanashi *et al.*, 1980). In other studies, six pyrrolizidine alkaloids and two related compounds — monocrotaline, lasiocarpine, petasitenine, senkirkine, clivorine, LX-201, viridefloric acid and pyrrole — were tested in the hepatocyte primary culture DNA-repair test, and compared with the results of an Ames test (Williams *et al.*, 1980). All six alkaloids were positive in the DNA-repair test system whereas all but monocrotaline had been found positive in the Ames test (Yamanaka *et al.*, 1979). These data are taken as an argument that the DNA-repair test has a better capacity than bacterial tests to detect genotoxic effects.

Mutagenic effects were also correlated with carcinogenic effects (Williams *et al.*, 1980). However, the two related substances which failed to induce mutations were not carcinogenic.

Among all the alkaloids tested in mammals, only three had previously been tested in *Drosophila* (Fig. 24): monocrotaline, lasiocarpine and heliotrine. Either in clastogenicity or in point mutation tests in hamster or in the hepatocyte primary culture DNA-repair test, these three alkaloids are in fact the most genotoxic, suggesting the real possibility of being able to extrapolate *Drosophila* data.

Nitrofurans

These compounds have been mostly utilized as antibacterial agents for local applications in human and veterinary medicines. They have also been used as food additives in the United States and in Japan (review of their mutagenicity in Tazima *et al.*, 1975).

In preliminary experiments, nitrofurantoin and nitrofurazone did not modify rat fertility (Jackson *et al.*, 1959). However, Zampieri and Greenberg (1964) and Waterbury and Freedman (1964) demonstrated a positive effect of nitrofurazone in bacteria. A comparable effect was also found for furazolidone by Szybalski (1958) and Waterbury and Freedman (1964). Experiments of McCalla (1965) and Woody-Karrer and Greenberg (1963) suggested a greater variation of response.

In other experiments, McCalla and Voutsinos (1974) investigated what kinds of modifications of molecular structures are related to modifications of mutagenic effects in *E. coli*. Although dealing with special strains (WP_2 and uvr A^-), these results already emphasize some interesting relationships between molecular structure and mutagenic activity in this class of molecule. These relationships might be exploited in practical work. First, the nitro group seems to be essential for mutagenic activity (Fig. 25). Substituted derivatives at position 9 in which a thiazolyl group is attached to the molecule show low or medium mutagenic activity. Clearly, their activity depends on the radical located at position 2 of the thiazolyl group. It seems that some steric considera-

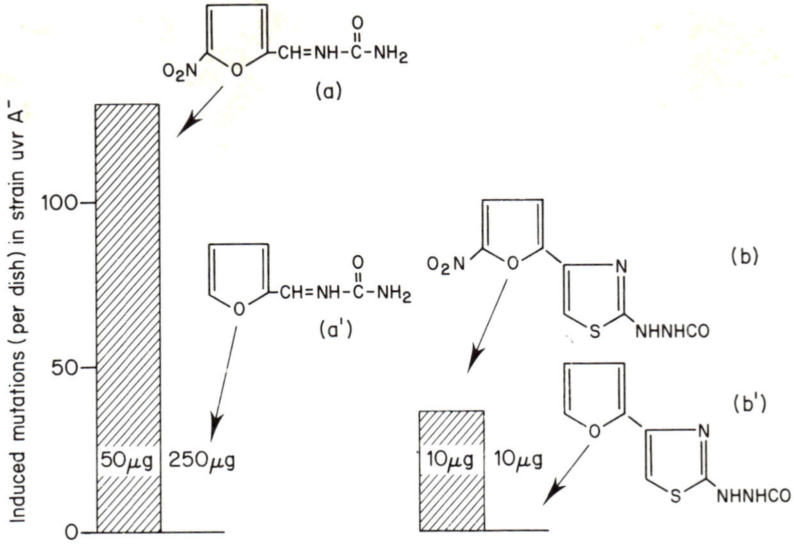

FIG. 25. Mutagenic efficiency of nitrofurans in *E. coli*. Derivatives with a nitro group only are mutagenic (After McCalla and Voutsinos, 1974.)

tions play an essential role since radicals that are too large decrease the activity (Fig. 26).

The compounds without a thiazolyl radical can be separated into three groups of strong, medium and no activity (Fig. 27).

Unfortunately, the classification of these compounds depends closely on the kinds of mutation taken as reference. Nevertheless, it can be seen that compounds which contain oxazolidinone or triazene rings are extremely mutagenic. In contrast, the presence of an aminohydantoin ring decreases the activity. Oxime and triazole radicals completely suppress the activity. In investigations with these compounds, it would be appropriate to vary the experimental conditions as much as possible, since paradoxically, in bacteria, some of them show less mutagenicity at increased concentrations. According to Ames *et al.* (1973), this relatively decreased activity when compared with the predicted mutagenicity is due to a stronger inactivation of important genes which are different from those of the test itself. All these data allow two conclusions to be drawn. First, new sets of experiments should be performed on the basis of other criteria of mutagenicity. Second, for practical purposes, the use would be indicated of substances having sufficient antibacterial power with a minimum mutagenic potential, e.g. derivatives without nitro groups, and the synthesis of molecules with lower mutagenicity recommended. On the other hand, Tazima *et al.* (1975) obtained positive mutagenic effects with three nitrofuran derivatives after treatment of silk worm oocytes.

Clastogenic effects of nitrofurans were detected in human lymphocytes by Tonomura and Sasaki (1973). They classified the compounds by order of

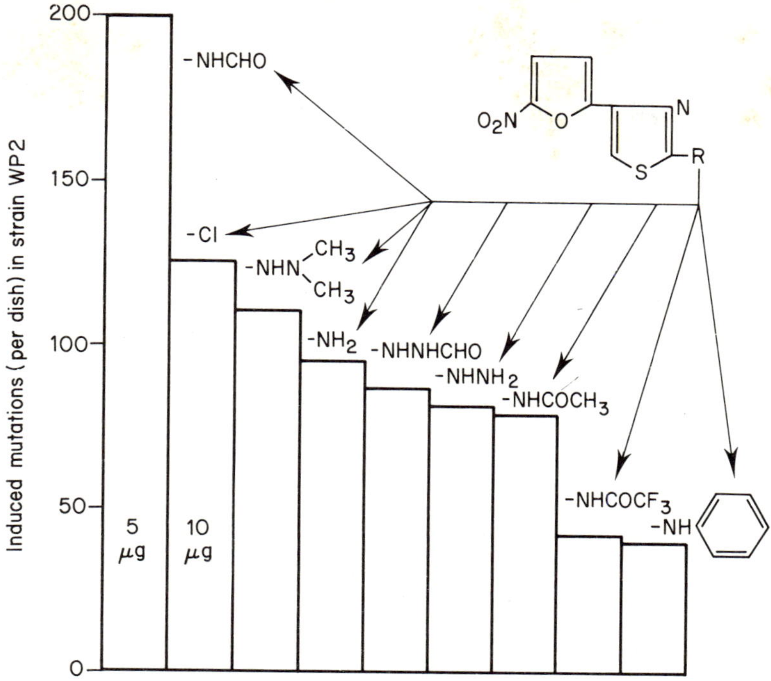

FIG. 26. Mutagenic efficiency of nitrofurans in *E. coli*.
Modifications of activity with radical R for compounds with a thiazolyl residue. (After McCalla and Voutsinos, 1974.)

decreasing activity as follows: furanizole, nitrofurylacrylamide, furpyrinole and furylfuramide (AF-2). In contrast, derivatives which possess an azomethine residue such as nitrofurazone, nitrofurantone and furazolidone, did not significantly increase the frequency of chromosomal aberrations.

Eight nitrofurans were more recently tested in Chinese hamster ovary cells cultured *in vitro* to detect modifications in the frequency of sister-chromatid exchanges, and the results were compared with the mutagenic activity in *Salmonella typhimurium* (Shirai and Wang, 1980).

All compounds tested increased to some extent the frequency of sister-chromatid exchanges, and there is a good correlation with the mutagenic activity found in *S. typhimurium*. There is also a fairly good correlation between sister-chromatid exchanges and clastogenicity. Thus, for nitrofurans, at least those in which a thiazolyl group is associated, the predictability derived from the relationship between structure and activity, based on steric considerations, is really noteworthy.

Aromatic amines

The mutagenic effects of two series of related amines were investigated in short-term tests (Shahin *et al.*, 1980a, b; survey in Shahin, 1982). The first

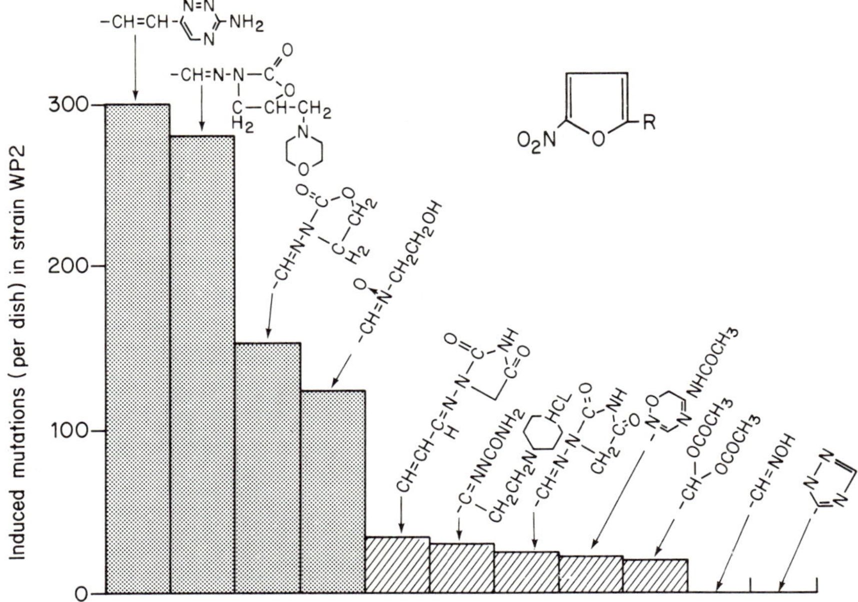

FIG. 27. Mutagenic efficiency of nitrofurans in *E. coli*. Modifications of activity with radical R of compounds without thiazolyl ring. Dotted areas: agents showing strong activity. Hatched areas: agents showing much lower activity. Two compounds at the right did not produce any activity (10mg per Petri dish). (After McCalla and Voutsinos, 1974.)

series comprised four derivatives of *m*-diaminobenzene (*m*-phenylenediamine) (*vide infra*). The mutagenic activity depended on the size of the substituting alkyl group at the C_1 position. When the size of this alkyl group was increased, the activity was decreased. In the second series, six diaminoalkoxybenzene compounds* were tested. In this series too, the mutagenicity was influenced by the size of the alkoxy group at the C_1 position. The highest mutagenicity was exhibited by the 2,4-diaminoanisole (methoxy derivative) but only after activation by microsomal enzymes. This is particularly important

NH2

R

NH2

m-Diaminobenzene

m-Diaminobenzene derivatives:

R = $-CH_3$, $-C_2H_5$, $-CH\genfrac{}{}{0pt}{}{CH_3}{CH_3}$, $-C_4H_9$

2,4 Diaminoalkoxy-benzene derivatives

R = $-O-CH_3$ (2, 4-diaminoanisole: positive in bacteria), $-O-CH_2-CH_3$, $-O-CH\genfrac{}{}{0pt}{}{CH_3}{CH_3}$,

$-O-CH_2-CH_2-CH_3$, $-O-CH_2-CH_2-CH_2-CH_3$, $-O-CH_2-CH_2OH$
(2, 4-diaminophenoxyethanol: negative in bacteria).

since this compound is used as a hair-dye (review in Loprieno *et al.*, 1982, see Chapter 4).

A model experiment was designed in rat (Shahin *et al.*, 1980a, b) to determine if, in conditions of topical application, mutagenic metabolites were detected in urine. Urine extracts actually showed mutagenic effects. This is not the case with other compounds such as 2,4-diaminophenoxyethanol which was negative.

Once more, the study of the relationship between structure and activity is relevant to the monitoring of populations i.e. to decide, on the one hand, which substance should be rejected and, on the other hand, in which direction harmless compounds should be sought.

Nitroimidazoles

There is a great variety of such compounds, all derivatives of the imidazole ring* The most widely used in medicine and also the best investigated for mutagenicity is metronidazole. Its antiprotozoan property has long been known, particularly against *Trichomonas vaginalis, Entamoeba histolytica* and *Giardia lamblia*, but also in the treatment of Crohn's disease. Nitroimidazoles have been tested in various test systems from bacteria to mammals (review in Voogd, 1981). Data are, however, somewhat fragmentary, except in bacteria where 47 compounds have been investigated. At present, relationships between structure and activity can only be derived from data obtained in bacteria. Three types of derivatives at position 2, 4 and 5 should first be distinguished. The 1-alkyl-2-nitroimidazoles are slightly more mutagenic than 1-alkyl-5-nitroimidazoles (Chin *et al.*, 1978) but the results are still contradictory. In the class of 1- or 5-nitroimidazoles, there is a clear relationship between reduction potential and mutagenicity (Wardman, 1977; Chin *et al.*, 1978). If a methyl group is attached to an atom of the imidazole ring located near the nitro group, the compound shows a strong activity. In contrast, if it is not located nearby, the activity is decreased; for example, 1,4-dimethyl-5-nitroimidazole is the most mutagenic compound of the series (Bauer et al., 1972) whereas 1,2-dimethyl-4-nitroimidazole is the least mutagenic (Berget and Weber, 1972). However, if there is an electron-negative group between the methyl group and the nitro group, the mutagenic activity is enhanced, as in the case of 5-chloro-1-methyl-4-nitroimidazole (Buttar and Siddiqui, 1980).

A particularity of the 5-methyl-4-nitroimidazoles is that when another methyl group is attached either at position 1 or 2 of the imidazole ring, the mutagenic activity is decreased so that these dimethylnitroimidazoles are only

```
                       R4 ——— N
                       ||     ||
* General formula     / \   /  \
                    R5    N     R2
                          |
                          R1
```

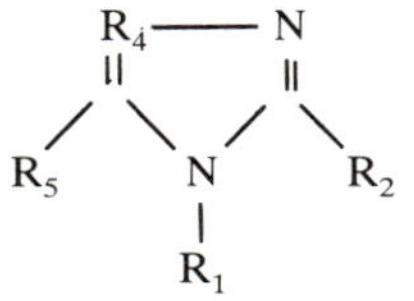

In metronidazole $R_1 = -CH_2-CH_2OH$
$R_2 = -CH_3$
$R_4 = -H$
$R_5 = -NO_2$

weak mutagens (Asquith *et al.*, 1974). As stated above, in test systems other than bacteria, i.e. yeast, fungi, *Drosophila* and mammals, the results for clastogenicity, micronucleus test, mutation assays and host-mediated assays are much less clear.

Additional questions need answering. It is well known that the metabolism of such compounds is quite different in mammals and in bacteria (review in Voogd, 1981). Another particularity worthwhile taking into account is the possibility of changing the effects under anaerobic conditions. With metronidazole, chromosome aberrations were observed in V79-399 Chinese hamster cells by incubation under anaerobic conditions (Korbelik and Horvat, (1980). Therefore, one can wonder if such anaerobic conditions are not occurring in human tissues. However, no increase in chromosome aberrations was observed in lymphocytes of patients administered the drug, at least for short-term tests (Hartley-Asp, 1979).

Another use of metronidazole, and sometimes other nitroimidazoles, is as a sensitizer to enhance the effects of ionizing radiations in tumour therapy where high serum concentrations should be reached (Dishe *et al.*, 1977). This sensitizing property should be kept in mind, for instance, in the case of X-ray examinations.

The research on nitroimidazoles, even if principally based on experiments on bacteria, has interesting applications. Even if it is not yet possible to replace metronidazole due to the positive risk–benefit balance, at least it is possible to restrict the use of such strongly mutagenic substances as 2-amino-5-(1-methyl-5-nitroimidazol-2-yl)-1,3,4-thiadiazole and 6-(2-dimethylaminoethoxy)-2-(5-nitro-1-methyl-2-imidazolyl-methylene)-1-tetralone sulphate.

Following the general principles outlined in this chapter, toxicologists are being increasingly required to investigate the variations in mutagenicity (positive or negative) generated by the modifications of the molecules of each chemical class. From some of the examples described above, it appears that metabolic studies should be systematically performed. After identification of metabolites mainly in blood or urine, simple knowledge of the rules governing the relationships between molecular structure and mutagenic activity could pilot future mutagenicity testing, and would save time for testing.

Chapter 6

Genetic Risks of Atomic Energy: a Model for Further Studies

> 'Radiation is but one of a number of dysgenic influences at work in human populations'
>
> Neel and Schull (1956)

Genetic effects of ionizing radiations are no longer to be demonstrated. Even in 1916, in epoch-making research, Muller clearly grasped the advantage of the use of X- or γ-rays as a tool in fundamental research to analyse genetic systems. In 1919 with Altenburg, he realized the role of mutations in the evolution of species.

However, slowly the idea spread that ionizing radiations represent a potential hazard for man due to the deleterious effects of various mutations (Muller, 1927). Radiations would not only be capable of increasing the number of inherited diseases, which would result in a heavy burden for human populations, but they could also lead eventually to genetic death (see below) on the basis of extrapolation from studies of animal populations. This research stressed the immediate need for man to control his own genotype. The rapid progress in the use of atomic energy for peaceful, or other, purposes amply strengthened this idea.

In what way are radiations harmful for genetic systems? Voluminous works have been devoted to this question (see Hollaender, 1954 in Gen. Refs).

Limiting the subject to the main points, one can roughly distinguish two kinds of effects. First, ionizing radiations act through energy dissipation within the chromosomes, either directly or indirectly via free radicals produced in living cells (see Bacq and Alexander, 1955 in Gen. Refs.; Stone, 1956). Second, radiations produce in the medium toxins capable of remaining for a rather long time, and of inducing long-term effects.

In genetic toxicology, we are generally concerned with low protracted doses of radiations, rather than with major accidents due to acute irradiations, which fall beyond the scope of genetics and demand special medical cures. Thus, what is essential is to investigate these chronic effects in order to assess their risks. Potential hazards of induced poisons should also be considered.

Several important problems demand our attention:

(1) Are the genetic effects of protracted, whole body exposure comparable with the same exposure given over a short period? In other words, are the effects of chronic doses comparable with the effects of acute doses at the same dose level?

(2) Can the genetic effects of low levels be evaluated by the same methods as the effects of higher levels?
(3) What would be the genetic consequences of a low exposure prolonged over several human generations?

There are different approaches to these problems. The first is to collect information from experiments on animal populations, e.g. *Drosophila* or mice. This is in fact the traditional approach, but extrapolation of the data to man remains difficult. To obtain more direct information the effects of testis irradiation were investigated in human volunteers, a procedure which raises ethical problems (Brewen and Preston, 1974). A third approach is to obtain information from the measurement of the DNA content of nuclei since there is a good correlation between mutation rate and DNA content (Abrahamson *et al.*, 1973). This is obviously a biased approach.

Practically, data intended to correlate doses and effects in man are collected in hospitals, where investigations are often fragmentary. Total mortality congenital malformations, infantile morbidity and sex ratio only allow an imprecise analysis. In the majority of cases it is not even possible to evaluate the genetic components of such pathological conditions. Nor is it possible to relate the frequency of a well-known inherited disease in a human population to the mean radiation dose given to this population, since all parameters which frame the genetic structure of a given population interact. The following parameters should be known: What proportion of the whole population is exposed to radiations and to what extent?

ESTIMATION OF THE GENETIC RISKS

Before answering this question, some comments on the effects of low-intensity irradiations are required. The effects of a chronic dose should be compared to the effects of the background level normally received by man during his whole life from cosmic rays, medical radioisotopes, X-ray examinations and, to a lesser extent, natural radioactivity. A scientific committee of the United Nations (UNSCEAR, 1972, in Gen. Refs.) estimated that the total average dose received by man up to the middle of his life (fixed at 30 years) is about 3 rads (i.e. 100 mrad/year). Correlatively, the frequency of major defects from genetic origin was estimated to be about 3%. This figure does not take into account dominant lethal mutations which would give rise to still-births but not transmitted to further generations. Nor does it take into account multiple minor mutations not recognized as such, or quantitative mutations (Chapter 10) which in the long run could modify the genetic structure of populations.

According to the data of Lüning and Searle (1971) in mouse, the dose that doubles the spontaneous frequency of mutations is of the order of 30 rads for acute irradiations by γ-rays and 100 rads for chronic irradiation at the testicular level. For radiations other than X-or γ-rays, e.g. neutrons, one should know the relative biological effectiveness, and in such cases doses would be given in milliroentgen (mR) per mass equivalent. According to Russel *et al.* (1958) and

Russel (1965), who measured the frequency of recessive mutations at seven specific loci in mice (Chapter 2), the average frequency per locus is 8×10^{-6} Vogel (1970) considers that in man the frequency of spontaneous mutations is of the same order of magnitude.

From the data obtained with human volunteers (Brewen and Preston, 1974) as well as from extrapolated data based on measurements of DNA content (Abrahamson *et al.*, 1973), it can be concluded that the frequency of mutations is two to three times higher in man than in mouse. Thus, 15 R would be a better estimate of the doubling dose. It should be kept in mind that these figures are derived from irradiations of spermatogonia, i.e. pre-meiotic stages, without knowing the effects on post-meiotic stages, e.g. spermatids, which might be more sensitive. Moreover, even when these calculations can be calculated in this latter case for point mutations and chromosome rearrangements, it is almost impossible to predict what would be the effects on the frequency of trisomies since it is not known in man to what extent ionizing radiations increase the non-disjunction rate except from indirect data on the increase of some human diseases in the progeny of exposed populations (see below).

On the basis of animal experiments, it can be expected that below a certain dose rate the effects are less marked, owing to the occurrence of repair processes at the level of the genetic code (see below).

Therefore, the second problem results from the difficulty of predicting the genetic damage at low doses of radiations using the methods at present available. According to Grahn (1972) this damage can be described in three different ways: (1) mutation rate per roentgen and per gene (as in *Drosophila* and mouse); (2) mutation rate per gamete; (3) the dose required to double the spontaneous mutation rate (see above).

Since the first two methods are uncertain due to our relatively poor knowledge of man's genetic system, the third has been preferred. But with this method another difficulty arises. According to Ehrenberg (1974), the notion of threshold — so useful in classical toxicology — is not applicable without restrictions in genetic toxicology. These limitations are not only valid for ionizing radiations, which are in some ways a general model, but also for chemical mutagens. In fact, in traditional toxicology, the threshold is generally clearly defined by the generally sigmoid shape of the dose–response curve. In contrast, in genetic toxicology, the dose–response relationship is generally linear because mutations under investigation are one-hit events. This dose–effect curve is of considerable importance in assessing genetic risks. This concept, well known for radiation, has been extended to monofunctional alkylating agents by Turtóczky and Ehrenberg (1969) and Osterman-Golkar *et al.* (1970). From these results it appears that extrapolation to low doses is imprecise, and that mutations could also be induced at doses below those that produce measurable effects (Ehrenberg, 1974).

Apart from those indicated above, are there other sources of information on the dose that doubles the mutation rate in human populations?

The only sources of human data in this matter come from Hiroshima and

Nagasaki atomic explosions, a few experiments on human volunteers and acute irradiation of patients. For various reasons, however, these data have only a limited bearing on genetics. Thus, the first generation born from irradiated populations might only show dominant mutations which according to plant and animal experiments are only a small proportion of all mutations actually induced. Even chromosome rearrangements could remain undetected for successive generations. In contrast, on the basis of the well-known principles of population genetics, it can be asserted that there is a real risk of recessive mutations spreading in the population (see next section).

Following the atomic explosions at Nagasaki and Hiroshima, the survivors were examined over a rather long period of time from 1946 to see if there were differences among the children of exposed and unexposed parents. This study was based on gross morphological criteria. No cytological analysis could be performed because no adequate method in mammals was available at that time. Definitive conclusions were difficult to draw. A shift in the sex ratio, indicative of sex-linked lethal mutations, was sought. The difference in the sex ratio between children from irradiated and unirradiated parents was not statistically significant (Schull and Neel, 1958), whereas significant differences do exist in the progeny of parents exposed to acute irradiations during therapy for diseases such as ankylosing spondylitis or malignant tumours (Lejeune *et al.*, 1960; Scholte and Sobels, 1964).

The frequency of trisomies resulting from failure of chromosome disjunction was slightly increased but only for sex chromosomes and chromosome translocations (Awa and Neriishe, 1972). In contrast, no autosomal trisomies were mentioned, whereas it is well known that the frequency of mongolism (Down's syndrome) which results from the trisomy of chromosome 21 is significantly enhanced after medical irradiations (Sigler *et al.*, 1965).

In further investigations, it was demonstrated that aberrant cell clones can persist for a very long time after the exposure. In this context, Sasaki and Miyata (1968) observed typical chromosome damage in lymphocytes of individuals exposed about 22 years before. The intensity of chromosome damage was clearly related to the distance from the hypocentre at the time of the bombing. The same conclusion can be extended to patients irradiated with acute doses (Bloom, 1972). These few examples show once more the difficulties of collecting pertinent data in human populations.

The answer to the third question requires a brief statement of a well-established concept which can be traced back to Muller's experiments (1950): genetic death.

GENETIC DEATH

According to the conception of Muller, if a whole population is irradiated for protracted periods over successive generations, genetic damage accumulates in this population. Even if the agent inducing the mutations has ceased to act for a long time, the investigated population would decay due to the accumulation of deleterious genes in homozygous carriers. The reason is that, in the carriers, these genes lead to death before the age of reproduction or alternatively to sterility. To demonstrate the reality of this sequence of events, it would be necessary to know the frequency in the population of genes of lethality, sublethality and subviability, i.e. the frequency of mutations which lead to precocious death (sometimes before birth), or which decrease fertility by various genetic mechanisms. These arguments have been supported by well-documented animal experiments.

In this context, ionizing radiations have been recommended and efficiently utilized for the biological control of insects (Wright and Pal, 1967, in Gen. Refs.; and Smith and von Borstel, 1972). In short, this procedure consists of collecting a sufficiently large sample of the insect population to be able to control and irradiate this sample at appropriate doses of ionizing radiations. X-rays and ^{60}Co γ-rays have been utilized for this purpose, and even neutrons of reactors have been suggested, though this is evidently unpractical. Doses should be sufficiently high as to induce more than one mutation per gamete but low enough not to alter the ability of males to reproduce. After irradiation, insects are released on their site. At well chosen doses, irradiated females are in general almost totally sterile due to the greater sensitivity of female sexual stem cells. In contrast, males remain able to mate and thereby introduce a lot of deleterious genes into the population. The invasion of the population by such genes will lead either to its rapid decay within a few generations or even to its completely dying out, especially when the selective pressure is superimposed on the effects of radiations. Control of the population size can be extended to successive generations.

If this procedure is adequately handled by man it will in some ways be more valuable than pesticides (Chapter 9). However, the ecological context should be carefully taken into account, and man should be particularly aware of the possibility of disrupting natural equilibria, leading to possible disasters.

This and other biological methods, that allow planned control of populations of insect vectors of disease is in some ways an application of the principle of genetic death after irradiation of a whole population at acute doses. This is in fact a 'sketch' of what could happen to a human population exposed to sufficiently high doses of a powerful mutagenic agent for successive generations.

How can this concept be extended to human populations submitted to low doses of radiation? Since from lower organisms to *Drosophila* and then to mammals there is in general an increase of radiosensitivity corresponding to an increase of genetic lethality, it is to be expected *a priori* that the human genetic system is even more sensitive than those of other mammals. What is the social meaning of these mutations? Intrauterine mortality is not followed by remote genetic consequences. Doubling the frequency of such mutations compared with their frequency at the equilibrium in a population would certainly result in a considerable social burden but would not necessarily mean genetic death. Examples of massive dominant lethality are frequent in animal and plant populations even when they are at genetic equilibrium. Thus, a certain proportion of lethal mutations can be frequently well tolerated in a population without leading inevitably to a disaster. In fact, one can to some extent rely on genetic defence reactions increasing the adaptability of the population towards deleterious factors. In fact, our knowledge of genetic death and adaptability in human populations should be improved, and new data based on more elaborate experimental models are expected. At present, the only way to proceed is to attempt to minimize the risks.

With the atomic age, however, a new line of research has developed. It aims to elucidate the fundamental protective mechanisms against radiations at the molecular level. In this respect the next questions should be answered: To what extent is chromosome damage repaired? and To what extent can we protect a genetic system?

REPAIR PROCESSES OF RADIO-INDUCED DAMAGE

The concept of repairing chromosome lesions, 'healing', can be traced back to Sax (1940, 1941). Wolff and Luippold (1956) distinguished several types of chromosomal lesions involving two types of repair processes. They suggested that the first type did not depend on metabolism, in contrast to the second. By fractionating the doses of γ-rays, Gilot-Delhalle *et al.* (1973) showed that ionic bonds interact in the fast repair processes of chromosome damage though the mechanisms involved in these processes are poorly understood. In contrast, the repair processes of the second type of lesion involve covalent bonds and require chemical energy, i.e. metabolism. Repair processes are different, at least quantitatively, in different species, and numerous factors can interact with these processes. Even in mammals, both quantitative and qualitative differences exist, and there is no general schedule directly applicable to man. Differences are located not necessarily in the genetic code itself, but also at the level of enzymes involved in repair processes and in a more general way at the level of metabolism as a whole.

What lesions can be repaired?

Since the research of Sax (1940, 1941), it became increasingly evident that the chromosomal lesions that can be observed after irradiation are only a small part of the total damage actually induced. This proportion has been estimated by various biased methods to be of the order of 10% (Lea and Catcheside, 1942). With other methods of calculation, comparable conclusions were reached for *Nigella damascena* (Ranunculaceae) chromosomes (Moutschen, 1968). After irradiation with ionizing radiations, and also after treatment with a large variety of chemicals, some chromosome regions other than chromosome constrictions are known to remain unstained or less stained. The true nature of such lesions, named 'gaps', is still unclear. They are generally thought to be primary lesions which were repaired but might in some cases undergo misrepair to give true chromosomal aberrations. Therefore, these lesions may be indicative of the total damage induced (review by Evans in Scott *et al.*, 1977).

At the molecular level it is well established that a special enzyme system — a ligase — restores the sequence of purine and pyrimidine bases. This process can repair only one strand linked to the complementary strand by hydrogen bonds. This reaction needs an adequate substrate and also a sufficiently powerful source of energy (generally ATP). Moreover, other more complex repair mechanisms still exist. In specific circumstances, it is known that several mutagenic agents — can induce thymine dimers. This is particularly the case after u.v. irradiation. Cells have two different mechanisms to deal with these lesions. In the first, endonucleases cut out the lesion, rather like surgeons do with an abscess or a tumour. The chemical details of these mechanisms are well understood in *E. coli* and there is no reason to think that they are very different in mammalian cells. This process, called excision-repair, works for only one DNA strand. Excising two strands simultaneously is seemingly lethal in the majority of cases. This first step of excision is followed by other events leading to repair. These are controlled by exo- and endonucleases, the role of which is in some way to fill the gaps left by the excision enzymes. This process is called non-conservative replication. It is still a matter of discussion whether it is catalysed by DNA polymerase present in all dividing cells or if other specific enzymes are involved. Whatever the chemical details, this process restores the nucleotide sequence.

This versatile mechanism operates not only in lower organisms but also in mammalian and human cells. In these latter cells it is complicated by the fact that the DNA is associated with histones resistant to nucleases, and this DNA^{-}histone complex has first to be dissociated before the repair process can be initiated.

Other, lesser known repair processes also occur in mammalian cells, including post-replication photoreactivation.

Post-replication repair operates within a few hours of the damage being induced. DNA replication is blocked, leaving some 'gaps' which are filled during *de novo* replication. Single strand exchanges may also occur. Photoreactivation exists to a limited extent in human cells and is specific for UV-induced damage in which pyrimidine dimers are formed (Fig. 28).

In mammals, all repair processes seem to be constitutive, i.e. of genetic origin. Another mechanism, known as inducible 'SOS' repair, occurs only in prokaryotes such as bacteria (Witkin, 1976; Sedgwick, 1976). It is far less efficient than the above mechanisms, leading to high mutation frequencies and becoming operative only when non-inducible repair processes are overloaded.

In several terrible inherited diseases, repair processes are altered. Models have been developed, on the basis of *in vitro* cultured cells of patients, to study the repair mechanisms at work after treatment with mutagenic agents and also in carcinogenesis and in ageing.

In the most well investigated disease xeroderma pigmentosum, the absence or low level of enzymes taking part in excision-repair processes provokes an extreme sensitivity to UV light. The incapacity of the cell to excise thymine dimers results almost inevitably in skin cancers (Cleaver, 1968, 1977). Patients

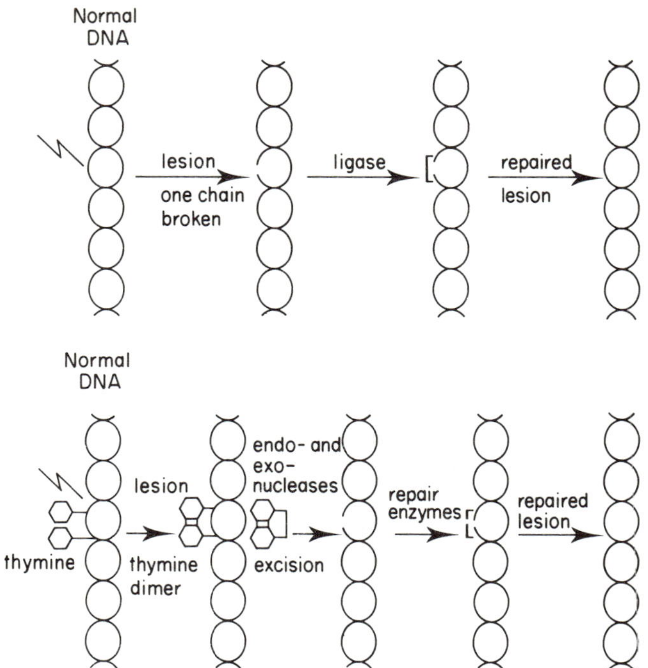

FIG. 28. Repair processes acting at the level of the genetic code in *E. coli*

suffering from the complex but fortunately rare syndromes such as Bloom's syndrome and Fanconi's anaemia, show a greater sensitivity to sunlight, other radiations or chemicals, and have a high risk of developing acute leukaemia. There is also a high frequency of chromosomal aberrations in some tissues. Patients suffering from ataxia telangiectasia develop lymphatic malignancy more frequently, are very sensitive to ionizing radiations and show chromosomal aberrations in lymphocytes and fibroblasts. In two strange pathological conditions — Cockayne's syndrome and progeria — an awful premature senility leading to death, sometimes before the age of 10 years, is observed in parallel with an exaggerated sensitivity to X-rays.

Without doubt, these still incurable diseases, are helping, and will certainly in the future contribute to our understanding of the biochemical defects responsible for the inaccuracy of repair processes, and will possibly help elucidate some fundamental mechanisms by which chromosomal aberrations are produced. It is also hoped that the better understanding of these processes will be helpful in curing such pathological conditions.

An important question in higher organisms is the relation between the damage observed at the molecular level as described above and the resulting chromosome breakage. In other words, how can a molecular lesion be transformed into a chromosomal aberration?

Theoretical models have been proposed, but none explaining the totality of the facts observed. It might be that the same aberrations are produced by more than one mechanism. Also the mechanisms are different for ionizing radiations and chemicals. The mechanisms described hitherto concern primary DNA damage, but eukaryotic chromosome is not merely DNA. Non-DNA components could also be damaged; for example, some agents could act indirectly by interacting with enzymes of DNA synthesis. These indirect mechanisms could be of environmental importance, and in this respect, many problems remain to be solved in mammalian cells. In Chapter 3 it was stated that some lesions result in losses of chromatin. The occurrence of such chromosome losses, especially small loses, does not mean *ipso facto* the immediate or deferred death of the cells in which they are observed. In fact, in such strongly buffered genetic systems as those of mammals, various regions of the genome can also have similar genic actions. Therefore, the destruction of one of these regions generally triggers compensation processes from the other. Regulating processes are in this case epigenetic, and are more complex than the preceding processes. Further details should be sought about these regulatory mechanisms.

MUTAGENIC POISONS PRODUCED BY IRRADIATION

Most of the potentially mutagenic molecules radio-induced in various media comprise peroxides, hydroperoxides, epoxides, on the one hand, and aldehydes and dialdehydes, on the other.

In specified conditions, depending on the dose of radiation and the nature of the irradiated substratum, other poisons can occur but less frequently. Although under usual irradiation conditions hydrogen peroxide is rapidly destroyed by catalase, a mutagenic action of this molecule has been described in lower organisms: *Neurospora* (Wagner *et al.*, 1950; Jensen *et al.*, 1951), *Staphylococcus aureus* (Wyss *et al.*, 1947, 1948) and *E. coli* (Demerec *et al.*, 1951). Chromosomal aberrations also have been observed in mouse ascites tumour (Schöneich, 1967).

Although the mutagenicity of the substances mentioned above is well documented (Chapters 4 and 5), the real problem is to know if, in irradiated substrata and under specific conditions of irradiation, the concentration of induced substance is sufficiently high to reach the threshold of mutagenic activity or to interfere with detoxification processes.

In this context, one application of atomic energy is food irradiation. Foods are irradiated for several purposes such as disinfestation of flour, inhibition of potato sprouting, food sterilization utilizing the bactericidal power of ionizing radiations (especially against, e.g., *Clostridrium botulinum* endospores, *Salmonella*). It is overt that under the technical conditions of irradiation no radioactive products are induced. On the other hand, it is firmly established in a large number of test systems that ingestion of irradiated food does not result in acute toxicity.

However, the possibility of diffuse cytotoxicity has not been completely ruled out for all foods because of the impossibility of testing all of them in all possible conditions. This situation prompted scientists to re-evaluate the methodology for mutagenicity testing and to make it more adequate for such kinds of investigations. There are several reviews on this subject (Scarascia-Mugnozza *et al.*, 1965; Spiher, 1968; Schubert, 1969; Kesavan and Swaminathan, 1971; Moutschen, 1973). Some include the problems caused by UV sterilization as well as the potential hazards of chemical techniques of sterilization. In these researches two approaches were outlined. For some researchers it seemed more logical to select simple compounds as experimental models, and then to increase the complexity of the models to show possible interactions. For others, it seemed more efficient and realistic to irradiate foods directly *in toto* under the conditions used in practice. Various foods were tested not only for mutagenicity, but also for teratogenicity and carcinogenicity. As simple models, irradiated carbohydrates were among the first tested since they occur in almost all foods (for a survey see Zelle and Hollaender, 1955; Scarascia-Mugnozza *et al.*, 1965).

Holsten *et al.* (1965) investigated the effects of sucrose, irradiated and then incorporated into the culture medium, on *Tradescantia* microspores, *Vicia* root-tip cells and *in vitro* cultured carrot callus. They described chromosomal damage comparable to that produced by low doses of radiations. Comparable effects were also reported by Shaw and Hayes (1966) in mammalian tissue cultures. In contrast, no effects were observed in *E. coli* WP 2 (tryptophan reverse mutations) and in *Salmonella typhimurium* (Watson and Schubert, 1969) for histidine revertants. Localized effects at specific chromosome regions were also reported in plant systems by Moutschen and Matagne (1965) after treatment with irradiated glucose at very high doses. This was confirmed by Ma (1968). On the other hand, after irradiation of sugar Schubert (1969) found some toxic molecules such as glyoxal, butyraldehyde and crotonaldehyde, sometimes in relatively large amounts. These latter substances are known to induce cytogenetic effects in mouse *in vivo* (Moutschen *et al.*, 1976), but at concentrations far above those produced by radiations.

Another application of irradiation is the irradiation of probands for animal laboratories, especially in experiments in which they need to be germ- or pathogen-free. Among irradiated foods, fruit juice and fruits, several sorts of flour, potatoes, milk powder, and various meats should be mentioned. All these irradiated foods were the subject of extensive research on many different organisms from phage to mammals (see Moutschen, 1973). Results were sometimes contradictory. If, on the other hand, the irradiation of complex media can give rise to toxic compounds in specified conditions (Schubert, 1969; Kesavan and Swaminathan, 1971), it is obvious, on the other, that, on the basis of the negative results obtained in so many studies, the mutagenic risks of irradiated foods *in toto* and in specified conditions should be considered negligible compared with the risks of the many compounds occurring everywhere.

As regards chronic exposure at low doses of ionizing radiations, much remains to be done to assess exactly the risks to man. It has been emphasized in Chapter 1–3 that no test system on its own can guarantee that no potential hazard has been omitted. New strategies should be adapted to the extreme diversity of the present situation.

In conclusion, the extensive research performed with ionizing radiations has been and will still be useful in the development of efficient experimental models in genetic toxicology and also to improve methodology.

Chapter 7

Hidden Mutagens

> 'They are ill-discoverers who think there is no land when they can see nothing but sea'
>
> F. Bacon

In Great Britain, in 1960, one hundred thousand turkeys given a diet containing peanuts died from a strange disease, the origin of which for a while remained completely unknown. For want of something better it was called 'Turkey X disease', a name which looks like a beautiful label on an empty bottle! One murder suspect was a microscopic fungus, the mould *Aspergillus flavus*. It was promptly realized, however, that by the time the poisoning of the animal had begun, the murderer had long left the scene of the crime. Nevertheless, he omitted to take his weapon with him: a terrible poison.

This short story illustrates the terrible tragedy of aflatoxin (Fig. 29). Entire colonies of rainbow trout exposed to this mycotoxin generally died from the same pathological condition, after developing liver cancer. Large-scale experiments on mammals, particularly on rats, have revealed the awful cytotoxic and carcinogenic properties of this fungal excretion product. Besides its toxicity, we can also mention its undoubted mutagenic activity. In *Neurospora*, 40 mg/l aflatoxin increases more than 200-fold the mutation rate at the adenine locus (*ad 3*) (Ong, 1970). However, it is not known which kinds of mutation the mycotoxin can induce in this test system, but from these experiments it can possibly be inferred that we are dealing with a 'single combat' between two toxic fungi. Its clastogenic effect has been pertinently demonstrated in *Vicia faba* (Lilly, 1965), in mammalian tissue cultures (Legator, 1966; Green *et al.*, 1967) and in cultured human leucocytes (Dolimpio *et al.*, 1968). Experiments in mouse (Epstein and Schafner, 1968) indicate a high frequency of dominant lethal mutations (for a general survey of mutagenic effects see Ong, 1975).

We are confronted here with a peculiar situation which somewhat resembles the situation caused by botulism. These bacteria, too, contaminate a medium (e.g. incorrectly prepared tinned food) without proliferating much, but excreting a sufficient amount of toxin to cause an acute alimentary problem.

Small amounts of aflatoxin, unable to induce detectable toxic effects, could reach or even overcome the threshold of mutagenic action. We are dealing here with a natural pollutant, produced incidentally and in quite special and unexpected conditions. Such substances deserve the name 'cryptomutagens' or hidden mutagens. Their detection is far from being as easy as in the case of aflatoxin, and raises difficult technical problems.

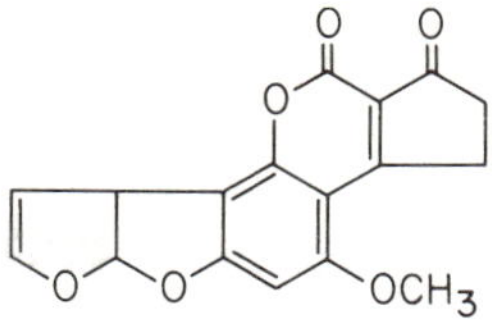

FIG. 29. Structure of aflatoxin B_1

We can distinguish five groups of hidden mutagens as follows:
(1) Chemical mutagens appearing incidentally in the environment independently from all kinds of human activity. Aflatoxin belongs to this group.
(2) Chemicals which by themselves have no mutagenic activity, but acquire some after transformation(s) in the environment in which they occur.
(3) Chemicals existing in the environment, either naturally or resulting from a human activity, but becoming mutagenic only after metabolic activation in the human body.
(4) Chemicals without any spontaneous mutagenic activity, but becoming mutagenic after successive transformations in the environment then in the human body.
(5) Chemicals without any spontaneous mutagenic activity, but possibly becoming mutagenic only after reaction(s) with another chemical incidentally introduced either in the environment or in the human body.

Chemicals of the first group principally include products of fungal or bacterial metabolism. On the one hand, chemicals of bacterial origin arising in soils are known to be particularly clastogenic (e.g. extracts of *Proteus*; Chapter 4). On the other hand, the usual or exceptional proliferation of various fungi which release into the environment many strange substances, some of which are beneficial to man (e.g. antibiotics!), has long drawn the attention of geneticists. In this context, we should also mention aflatoxins from several fungal species such as *Aspergillus flavus, Aspergillus parasitus* and *Penicillium pulverulum*, ocratoxin (from *Aspergillus ochraceus*), sterigmatocystin (from *Aspergillus versicolor, nidulans* and *bipolaris*), aspertoxin (from *Aspergillus flavus*), zearalenone (from *Fusarium graminearum*), and also many other molecules for which information about their mutagenicity is not always available (Fig. 30).

The risk of massive contamination is not great in as much as the foods are conserved in good condition. The recent finding of toxins in *Penicillium roqueforti*, a component of Roquefort cheese, is more disturbing. A terrible toxin called PR (for *Penicillium roqueforti*) was isolated and found to be lethal for rats at low doses (Wei *et al.*, 1973, 1975). Two classes of molecules could be identified. One, belonging to the group of eremofortins, was investigated to establish relationships between the chemical structure and biological properties (Moulé *et al.*, 1977, 1980). The genetic effects of this family of toxins were thoroughly investigated in the eukaryotic organisms: *Saccharomyces cerevisiae* and *Neurospora crassa*, and they were found to induce reverse

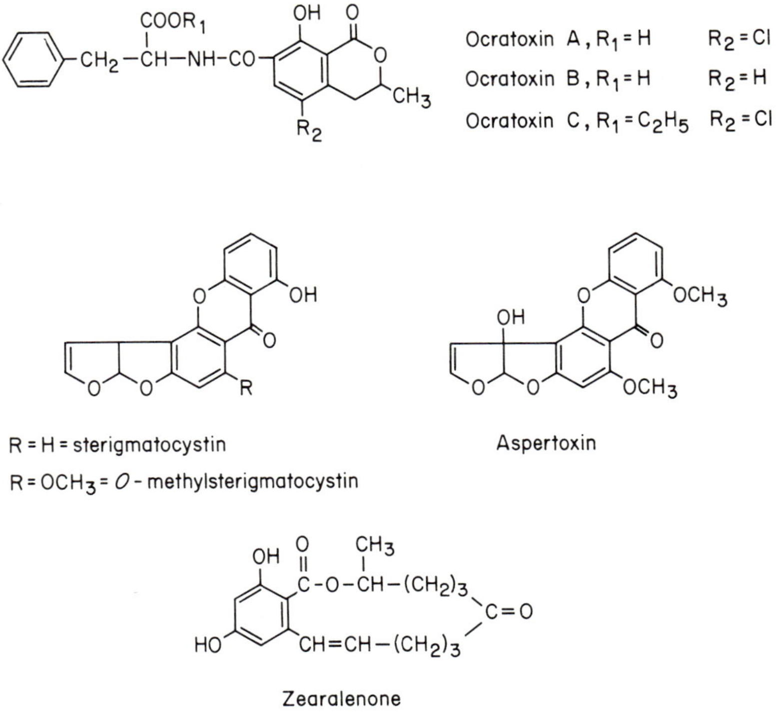

Ocratoxin A, $R_1 = H$ $R_2 = Cl$
Ocratoxin B, $R_1 = H$ $R_2 = H$
Ocratoxin C, $R_1 = C_2H_5$ $R_2 = Cl$

R = H = sterigmatocystin
$R = OCH_3$ = *O*-methylsterigmatocystin

Aspertoxin

Zearalenone

FIG. 30. Formulae of some mutagenic substances produced by lower organisms in specific conditions

mutations, conversion and somatic crossing-over under specific experimental conditions (Wei *et al.*, 1979) without metabolic activation.

Another mycotoxin, botryodiplodin, initially found in another fungus, was also detected in *Penicillium roqueforti*. It was mutagenic in *Salmonella typhimurium* (TA 98) in the histidine reversion test without metabolic activation (Moulé *et al.*, 1981a). Effects on mammalian cells, in which it inhibits cell growth and alters DNA, RNA and protein syntheses, were described (Moulé *et al.*, 1981b). How dangerous is the presence of such poisons? The risk should not be exaggerated since they were detected only in a very limited number of strains, and normally being absent from the cheese. However, since mutation towards a producing strain is always a possibility, the cheese should be permanently controlled.

Analogues of purines and pyrimidines have also been mentioned as substances released by fungi (Chapter 4). It could be that the mutagenicity of such kinds of chemicals, which have not been extensively investigated from the viewpoint of genetic hazards, is higher than expected and that secondary unsuspected effects might be detected. Classical tests of mutagenicity could possibly solve this problem simply. Several chemicals can acquire mutagenic properties in the environment, thereby raising more complicated questions.

For some years, a somewhat unstable chemical, diethylpyrocarbonate

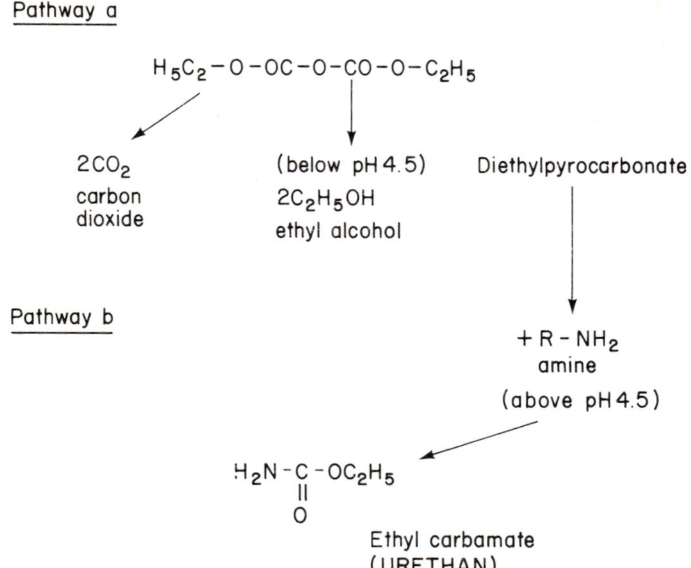

FIG. 31. Chemical transformations of diethyl pyrocarbonate (Baycovin)

(Baycovin), has been added to some alcoholic beverages to make them effervescent or as an antibacterial agent. This compound is not mutagenic, and usually splits into two molecules of alcohol and carbon dioxide. However, when the acidity of the solution is not too strong (above pH 4.5) and when amines or amino groups are available in the medium, the reaction of the compound follows a quite different pathway (Fig. 31, pathway b), giving rise to ethyl carbamate, better known as urethan. This pharmaceutical is well known by cancerologists who still use it as an antileukaemic agent. Its high antimitotic activity is in itself sufficient to warrant caution. For a long time it was thought that the amount of poison was too low to exert any effect. However, extensive investigations by Löfroth and Gejvall (1971) and Fischer (1972) revealed that the amount of urethan produced was far from being negligible. This observation underlines the necessity of using sufficiently powerful techniques to detect mutagens in the environment. According to these data, the threshold of mutagenic action is reached.

Clastogenic effects of this substance on plant cells had previously been demonstrated by Oehlkers (1943, 1953). Numerous experiments were performed on bacteria, *Drosophila* and mammals (for a review see Bateman, 1976), but the results of these experiments remain contradictory. Bateman (1967) did not find an increased frequency of dominant lethal mutations in mice. It is possible, therefore that the threshold of action for these mutations, mainly of the chromosome class, had not been reached. New experiments are needed. It is not completely ruled out that urethan could be first transformed into *N*-hydroxyurethan, which acts as an alkylating agent.

In contrast, according to Freese *et al.* (1968), urethan would react with DNA only after the formation of peroxide radicals, and would therefore belong to the second group of hidden mutagens (see below). Recently, urethan was shown to induce tissue-specific effects in mammals, such as sister-chromatid exchanges, but only after *in vivo* administration in bone marrow, liver and spermatogonial cells (Roberts and Allen, 1980).

Other substances have the dangerous property of being transformed into active mutagens in the body. Usually, the human body is extraordinarily equipped to detoxify a large variety of compounds. But beside these physiological detoxification processes, activation processes also occur.

According to Peters (1952, in Gen. Refs.) conception, the body undertakes in such cases a kind of 'lethal synthesis'. In the present context, we are not dealing, properly speaking, with 'lethal syntheses' but with what we could call 'mutagenic syntheses'. In these activation processes, two conditions are of importance: a sufficiently fast transformation without reaching the toxicity level and then a sufficient accumulation of the transformed compound in the gonads where it can show mutagenic activity.

Two additional questions arise: How to identify the transformed metabolite(s)? and How to evaluate the period during which it remains active?

Metabolic activation can occur in microsomes of the liver cells for most nitrosamines and cyclophosphamides. The formation of mutagenic compounds after interaction with these cell organelles was investigated by Malling (1971) for dimethylnitrosamine. Vogel *et al.* (1973) showed that triazenes belong to a relatively new group of mutagens with an indirect action (Table 5). Some of these molecules (Fig. 32) are transformed into formaldehyde by the enzymatic microsomal fraction which contains NADPH. In this way, they become potential alkylating agents as already suggested by the work of Preussmann (1968, 1969) and Preussmann *et al.* (1969).

N-Hydroxylation, a detoxification process frequently occurring in many pesticides, can form mutagenic molecules in the body. According to Freese *et al.* (1968), many pharmaceuticals synthesized from hydrazine (isocarboxazid, nialamide, phenelzine, as well as isonicotinic acid hydrazide or Rimifon) react in the body — maybe outside the body in specific conditions — with oxygen to produce hydrogen peroxide or peroxide radicals. Therefore, it is not surprising that some clastogenic properties of these substances have been identified (Chapters 4–6).

Röhrborn *et al.* (1972) made the peculiar observation that isoniazid shows some mutagenic effects in the host-mediated assay, but paradoxically not in the dominant lethal mutation test. The interpretation of these results is not quite clear. It could be suggested that a sufficiently high concentration of the metabolized substance to induce mutations is not reached in the gonads. One could also suggest a detoxification pathway that is quite different or faster in the gonads. Finally, a higher sensitivity of the micro-organisms used in the host-mediated assay could provide another plausible explanation. It is therefore necessary to correlate the effects directly observed in sex cells with the effects obtained in micro-organisms. These examples suffice to show that the

1 C_6H_5—N=N—N(CH_3)$_2$

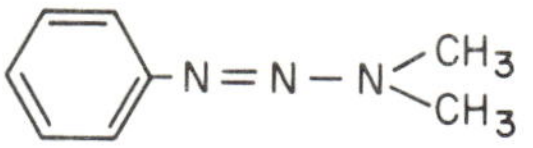

1-Phenyl-3,3-dimethyltriazene (PDT)

2 C_5H_4N—N=N—N(CH_3)$_2$

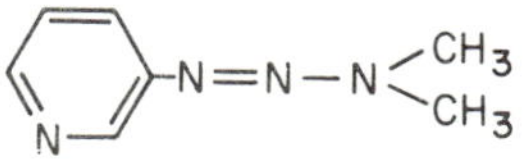

1-(Pyridyl-3)-3,3-dimethyltriazene (PyDT)

3 O←NC_5H_4—N=N—N(CH_3)$_2$

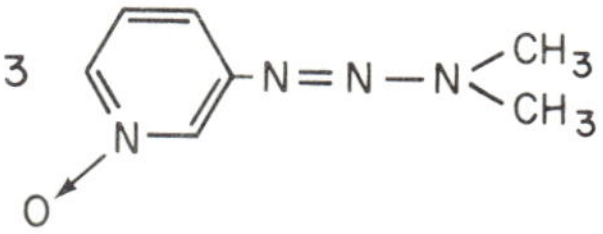

1-(Pyridyl-3-*N*-oxide)-3,3-dimethyltriazene (PyNDT)

FIG. 32. Formulae of three triazenes used in experiments (results briefly reported in Table 5)

metabolism of all suspected substances is a first step to take into account, keeping in mind: (1) that all data on mammalian metabolism do not *ipso facto* replace a detailed investigation in man;
(2) that man himself can possess diverse metabolic pathways.

Some situations are sometimes made complex because a compound can act through different mechanisms at one and the same time. In this respect, captan (Fig. 33, model 1) commonly used as fungicide could act mainly after metabolic transformation. It is well demonstrated that its toxicity in fungi is due to a reaction with the sulphydryl classical bonds (—SH groups) of some important cell constituents (maybe also with other chemical groups such as —OH, —NH_2 or —COOH). Owens and Novotny (1959) thought that the toxicity was due to the molecule itself prior to transformation; but Lukens and Sisler (1958) thought, conversely, that the condensation of captan with sulphydryl-containing molecules was followed by decomposition into the active moiety (Fig. 33, model 2). In this context, these researchers suggested that, in *Saccharomyces pastorianus*, the thiophosgene formed by decomposition is the main toxic agent. Is it the same situation concerning genetic effects?

The mutagenic potential of captan has been described in *E. coli* and in mammalian cells cultured *in vitro* (Legator and Verrett, 1967). To understand the mechanism(s) of action of this fungicide, it would be necessary to investigate the action of each metabolic product supposed to be mutagenic and the metabolic modifications at increased doses. The mutagenic effects of captan and related compounds have been reviewed by Bridges (1975).

For more than a decade the idea grew that it might be easier to show

TABLE 5. Genetic effects of three triazenes in various organisms

Organisms	Criteria	Effects*			Authors
		PDT	PyDT	PyNDT	
Neurospora crassa	Forward mutation at *ad 3* locus	+++	not investigated	not investigated	Ong and de Serres, 1971
Saccharomyces cerevisiae	Gene conversion at *ad 2* and *irp 5* loci	++	+	−	Fahrig, 1971
Saccharomyces cerevisiae (host-mediated assay)	Same criteria	++	+++	+++	Fahrig, 1971
Drosophila melanogaster	Dominant lethal	+++	0	0	Vogel, 1971
	Recessive lethal mutations	+++	+	+++	Vogel, 1971
Human leucocytes	Chromosome damage	±	±	±	Vogel *et al.*, 1973

* PDT = 1-phenyl-3, 3-dimethyl triazene; PyDT = 1-(pyridyl-3)-3, 3-dimethyl triazene; PyNDT = 1-(pyridyl-3N-oxide)-3, 3-dimethyl triazene.

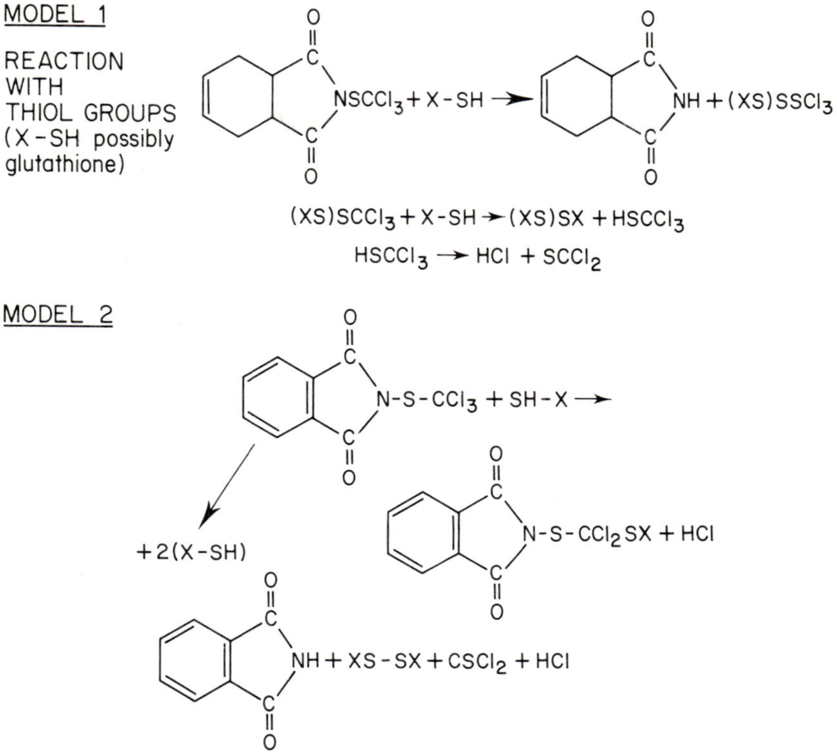

MODEL 1

REACTION WITH THIOL GROUPS (X-SH possibly glutathione)

$NSCCl_3 + X\text{-}SH \rightarrow NH + (XS)SSCl_3$

$(XS)SCCl_3 + X\text{-}SH \rightarrow (XS)SX + HSCCl_3$

$HSCCl_3 \rightarrow HCl + SCCl_2$

MODEL 2

$N\text{-}S\text{-}CCl_3 + SH\text{-}X \rightarrow$

$N\text{-}S\text{-}CCl_2SX + HCl$

$+2(X\text{-}SH)$

$NH + XS\text{-}SX + CSCl_2 + HCl$

FIG. 33. Mechanisms of action of captan (*N*-(trichloromethylthio)-4-cyclohexene-1, 2-dicarboximide)

metabolic activation in *in vitro* test systems than *in vivo*. Short-term tests would obviously permit the screening of a much larger number of suspected compounds within a shorter time.

From a symposium on the role of metabolic activation in producing mutagenic and carcinogenic environmental chemicals, some important conclusions emerged (de Serres *et al.*, 1976, in Gen. Refs.). One problem is to extrapolate the *in vitro* data to the *in vivo* situation. Malling (1966) suggested comparing the results obtained with bacterial tests, with and without microsomal enzymes, with the results of the host-mediated assay. It would be a way to validate the *in vitro* model. However, in spite of significant metabolic differences between mammalian tissues, short-term tests such as the *Salmonella*-microsome Ames test allowed mutagens and carcinogens to be detected. This is an important conclusion since the list of compounds that require metabolic activation before becoming mutagenic is growing fast.

After nitrosamines and cyclophosphamide, aflatoxins were found to be activated as well as polycyclic hydrocarbons. These latter compounds have long been known for their carcinogenic properties. It has been reasonably demonstrated that they are first converted into electrophiles before becoming active. Then polycyclic hydrocarbons displayed mutagenicity in the Ames test (Ames, 1976), from which the relationship mutagen–carcinogen was inferred. Once more, researchers endeavoured to link mutagenicity with carcinogenicity, sometimes raising more problems than they solved.

Activation processes are ubiquitous. About a decade ago, activation of promutagens to mutagens was noticed in higher plants. It was made clear by the observation that a widely used herbicide belonging to the *s*-triazine group, atrazine (2-chloro-4-ethylamino-6-isopropylamino-*s*-triazine), increased the frequency of *waxy* mutants in maize (Plewa and Gentile, 1976a). On the other hand, it was not mutagenic in microbes (references quoted in Adler, 1980). Therefore, the mutagenic activity is due to a metabolite arising in plant tissues. Hence the idea to prepare plant microsomal fractions to activate atrazine into an ultimate mutagen. This approach was rewarding since atrazine added to a medium supplemented with plant microsomal fractions proved to be mutagenic in *E. coli* and *S. typhimurium* (quoted in Plewa and Gentile, 1982), convertogenic at the loci *trp 5* and *ade 2* of *Saccharomyces cerevisiae* strain H 201/4.4 (Plewa and Gentile, 1975, 1976b). A total of 32 pesticides were tested in the same way; five were actually plant-activated (Gentile and Plewa, 1981).

Even if such agricultural compounds do not seem to have adverse effects on mammalian cells, according to a preliminary report (Chollet *et al.*, 1982), plant activation of such compounds into mutagens and the possible accumulation of these mutagens in crops is a potential hazard for the consumer which should be considered by government agencies. Fortunately many substances are not activated by plant microsomal fractions, but are in contrast deactivated. This is so for strong alkylating agents such as *N*-methyl——nitrosourea (Yano, 1979) and ethyl methanesulphonate (Scott *et al.*, 1978). Such fractions also detoxify tryptophan pyrolysates (Chapter 4). Since they are heat- and pronase sensitive their proteinic nature was suggested (Kada *et al.*, 1978; Morita *et al.*, 1978). The finding of activation processes in plants open a new chapter of genetic toxicology, leaving more room for hidden mutagens. Metabolic differences between plant and animal kingdoms need to be investigated, especially for agricultural compounds.

Among the chemicals that are transformed in the environment and then in the human body, nitrates and nitrites occupy a prominent place. Although their antibacterial efficiency is low, they are still used to preserve meats, fish and cheese. Nitrates can be reduced to nitrites by bacteria in the oesophagus and stomach. On their own, nitrites are directly utilized to enhance and to fix the colour of meats by decomposition into nitric oxide which reacts with the iron of haemoglobin and stabilizes it as methaemoglobin. It is precisely to this reaction with haemoglobin that the high toxicity of nitrites is due, especially in children. If the whole amount of added nitrites reacts, a noxious effect is not expected to occur. Unfortunately, this is not the case when there is an unreacted excess. When the acidity of the medium is sufficiently high (below pH 4) nitrites react giving nitrous acid. This reaction which can already occur in meat will certainly also occur in the highly acidic stomach contents (pH 1.1).

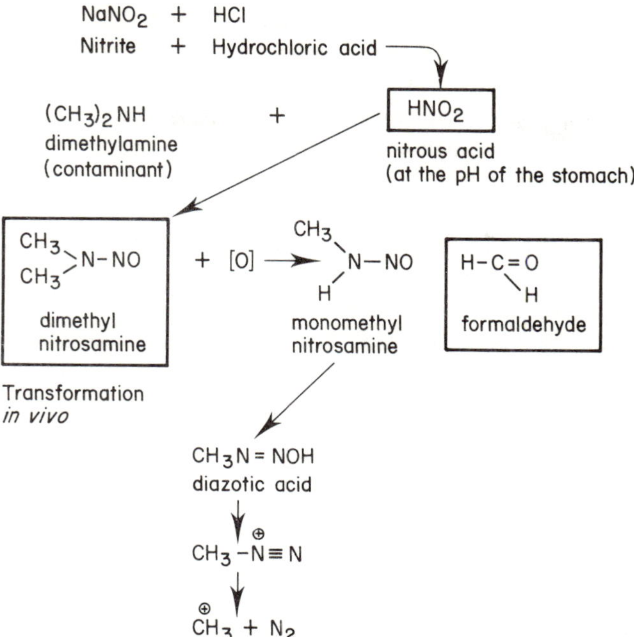

FIG. 34. Production of mutagenic molecules by nitrites

The mutagenic effects of nitrous acid are well known.

For technical reasons, the genetic effects of nitrites have been almost exclusively investigated in lower organisms (e.g. *Escherichia coli, Salmonella typhimurium, Neurospora crassa, Saccharomyces cerevisiae*, etc), even at the molecular level (tobacco mosaic virus, *Pneumococcus* transforming factor and also *Bacillus subtilis* and *Haemophilus*) (references in Fishbein *et al.*, 1970, in Gen. Refs.), and similar research is needed in higher organisms. But this is only the first tier of a more complicated scaffolding! In a second step, nitrous acid* can react with dimethylamine almost always present in the medium (especially in meat) giving rise to a nitrosamine** and formaldehyde (Fig. 34). We are already familiar with this latter intruder (Chapter 4). In contrast, nitrosamines deserve careful examination. The ubiquitous occurrence of such molecules is more alarming, though some researchers still consider the presence of dimethyl- and diethylnitrosamine here as an artifact (Eisenbrand *et al.*, 1981). They could practically be classified in each of our major subdivisions in Chapter 4.

Beside their formation from nitrites by reaction with amines occurring even at low temperature, nitrosamines can be found independently from this reaction in a great variety of foods such as smoked fish, smoked meat, some edible mushrooms as well as in cigarette smoke. We have already mentioned in

* It has been shown that this substance is highly reactive (Lijinsky, 1974).

** One of the compounds formed in such reactions could as well be ethylnitrosourea, one of the most potent mutagenic agents for, e.g., mammalian spermatogonia (Russel *et al.*, 1979).

this chapter that nitrosamines transformed in the body can form mutagens. According to Lijinsky *et al.* (1968), we are dealing with molecules capable of methylating DNA guanine into 7-methylguanine, a crucial step in the production of mutations. There are even strange conditions under which nitrosamines can be formed. For instance, dimethylnitrosamine occurs in urine following reaction with dimethylamine during bladder infections with bacteria such as *Proteus* (Radomski *et al.*, 1978). It was considered responsible for some bladder cancers, but it has since been shown using labelled molecules in rat that a large proportion of dimethylnitrosamine formed in the bladder diffuses into the peripheral circulation (Hill *et al.*, 1973).

Thus it could also be responsible for other cancers, including liver.

Although no mutagenic effects of several nitrosamines remained undetected in various lower organisms (*Escherichia coli*: Geissler, 1962; Podogina, 1966. *Serratia marcescens:* Geissler, 1962. *Saccharomyces cerevisiae* and *Neurospora crassa*: Marquardt *et al.*, 1964), they were found to induce reverse mutations at the locus *ad 3B* (Malling, 1966) in *Neurospora crassa*.

Genetic effects of dimethylnitrosamine in *Drosophila* had formerly been mentioned by Rapoport (1948) (see also Rapoport, 1966), and for dimethyl- and *N*-butylmethylnitrosamine by Pasternak (1962, 1963, 1964). For *N*-diethyl-*N*-nitrosamine and *N*-ethyl-*N*-nitrourethan, Fahmy *et al.* (1966, 1968) described anomalies of chromosome disjunction in *Drosophila* as well as various lesions (including translocations), recessive lethal and visible sex-linked mutations and also crossing-over modifications.

In *E. coli*, Sd 4, Hussain and Ehrenberg (1974) investigated the mutagenicity of methyl-, ethyl- and isopropylamine alone and in combination with sodium nitrite. The two first substances in combination with sodium nitrite are significantly mutagenic while isopropylamine plus sodium nitrite does not induce a detectable frequency of mutations higher than that occurring with the nitrite alone.

Veleminsky and Gichner (1968) compared the efficiency of the molecules of this group in *Arabidopsis thaliana* (Fig. 35). On the basis of the criteria selected, it seems that, in this organism, a methyl group is needed to confer mutagenic activity, except for ethylvinyl derivatives.

Investigations by Gabridge and Legator (1969) on host-mediated assay after injection of *Salmonella typhimurium* as marker, showed mutagenic effects of nitrosamines in this organism. Doses ranging from 20 to 50 mg/kg yielded positive results. Results in directly treated mammals are expected.

To summarize, we are dealing here with a series of complex reactions (Fig. 34). This complex problem has been recently reviewed (Hartman, 1982). Some chemical reactions such as oxidoreductions can form nitrites in the environment. Independently, nitrosamines can arise by quite different routes. In the body, these molecules follow a long chain of reactions which can eventually lead to a sufficiently high concentration of the substance in the gonads to induce irreversible damage.

Another adverse effect of nitrites illustrates the fifth category in which two

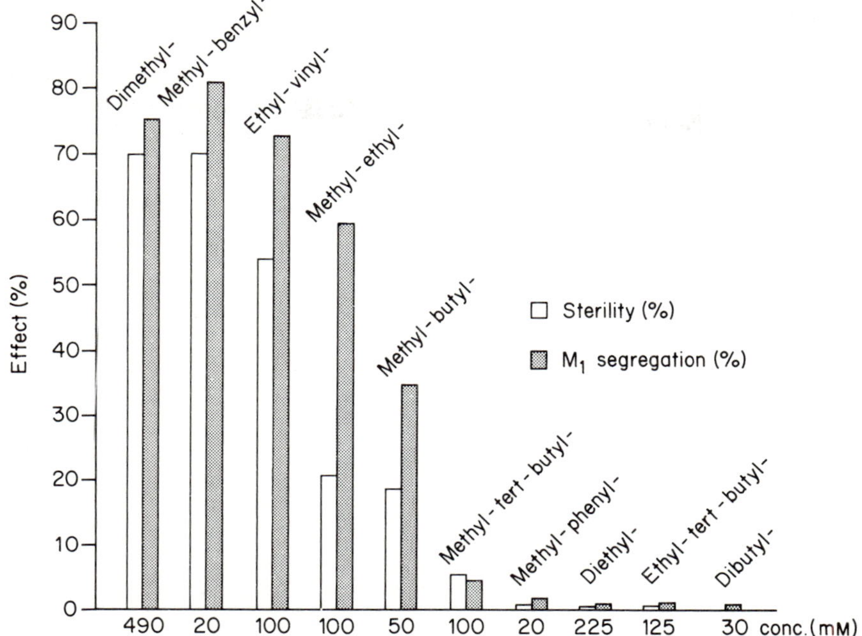

FIG. 35. Comparison of genetic effects of nitrosamines in *Arabidopsis thaliana* (Cruciferae). (After Veleminsky and Gichner, 1968.)

substances of completely independent origins react together in the body to give rise to a true mutagen. In this context, a group of researchers from Oak Ridge advised the American population against the effects of the insecticide carbaryl (Sevin) (Elespuru *et al.*, 1973). In itself, this substance has a low toxicity and is efficiently eliminated by the body. However, it reacts with nitrites present in excess in food and is transformed into nitrous acid in acidic media. Thus, nitrosocarbaryl can be formed in the stomach by reaction of two compounds of different origins. This substance is an analogue of nitrosomethylurethan, the mutagenicity of which has been demonstrated in two bacteria: *Haemophilus influenzae* and *Escherichia coli*.

From these data it was concluded that carbaryl is a more powerful mutagen than nitrosomethylnitroguanidine, which is one of the most mutagenic substances known so far. The risk is high if one thinks of the frequent use in various countries of carbaryl as an insecticide for spraying fruits, legumes, and fodder, some economically interesting crops and for the disinfestation of poultry and other domestic animals.

The basic chemical group common to all these substances and other insecticides should, for the same reasons, be considered potentially mutagenic. A few interactions between molecules belonging to remote chemical classes and resulting in mutagenic syntheses in the body have been described in the literature. It is not necessary to give many examples to draw attention to the importance of potential mutagens.

The notion of hidden mutagens underlines the necessity of considering genetic hazards as a whole on the level of the biosphere. This will be the subject of Chapter 9, This is not the time for 'witch hunts' but to attempt to detect lucidly and systematically all the potential hazards that surround us.

Chapter 8

Problems Raised by Cumulative Effects

'Singulière fortune où le but se déplace
Et, n'étant nulle part, peut être n'importe où!'

Ch. Baudelaire: *Le Voyage*
(Les fleurs du mal)

Up to now, we have attempted to detect everywhere in the environment, factors with potential genetic effects with reference to methods which allow them to be identified. This procedure is, in general, too analytical since in his environment man is rarely exposed only to one agent at one time.

In contrast, experimental results on genetic effects have been obtained with mammals systematically treated in optimized conditions.

In his daily life, however, man does not enjoy such a privilege. We are all the time confronted by multiple parameters. In short, three main possibilities occur:

(1) The same substance can be taken up several times. A single dose would not cause any problem, but after repeated doses there is a possibility of the threshold of mutagenic activity being reached or even surpassed.

(2) The presence of a 'cofactor' in the environment completely changes the mutation spectrum, thus transforming a harmless substance into a dangerous mutagen. This sequence is somewhat similar to that for hidden mutagens described in Chapter 7.

(3) The most frequent possibility occurs when numerous mutagenic agents act together, either when part of the same environment (e.g. food, water, air, pharmaceuticals, cosmetics, pesticides), or when arising from different sources.

More complex possibilities exist in which several factors are intertwined. In all these cases, it is well demonstrated that mutagenic agents from the same or different classes can interact, possibly resulting in synergistic effects. In contrast, there are examples of mutagenic substances having antagonistic effects (Chapter 10). The more powerful the chemicals (e.g. pesticides or chemotherapeutic agents), the more frequent are the synergistic effects. Organomercury compounds would seem to be typical of substances with multiple risks, and their toxic, mutagenic and clastogenic effects have been amply investigated (review in Léonard *et al.*, 1983). Previously, Kostoff (1939, 1940) described for the first time colchicomitotic effects of ethylmercury chloride in a fungicide mixture. Mineral salts of mercury have also some colchicomitotic potential, comparable to organic derivatives (Fahmy, 1951;

Degraeve, 1967). Somatic mutations were induced in plants (MacFarlane, 1950). Ramel and Magnusson (1969) pertinently demonstrated the clastogenic potential of organomercury compounds. In a first series of experiments, onion roots were treated with six different compounds: Panogen 5, Panogen 8, methylmercury dicyandiamide, methylmercury hydroxide, phenylmercury hydroxide and methoxyethylmercury chloride. Some data on the effects of such compounds are given in Table 6.

TABLE 6. Effects of a 72-h treatment of onion root-tip chromosomes with organomercury derivatives. (Ramel, 1969)

Substance	Minimal dose which produces colchicomitotic effects		Highest dose without cytological effects	
	mol/l × 10^{-7}	ppm Hg	mol/l × 10^{-7}	
Panogen 5*	2.5	0.05	1.9	0.04
Panogen 8*	8.0	0.16	3.2	0.06
Methyl mercury dicyandiamide	6.0	0.13	2.5	0.05
Methyl mercury hydroxide	8.0	0.16	2.0	0.04
Phenyl mercury hydroxide	8.0	0.16	4.0	0.08
Methoxyethyl mercury chloride	31.4	0.63	16.0	0.32

* Compounds known under the name Panogen (e.g. Morsodrin, Panodrin A 13, Panterra, Pandrinox) are pesticides containing methylmercury dicyandiamide as active component.

formula $CH_3{-}Hg{-}N(H){-}C({=}NH){-}NC{\equiv}N$

According to Ramel (1969), these results emphasize the fact that the confidence limit between the highest concentrations at which no effect can be detected and the lowest concentrations at which colchicomitotic effects are observed is quite narrow.

Clastogenic effects have also been found after treatment with halogenated organomercury compounds (Fiskesjö, 1969). Moreover, other experiments of Ramel and Magnusson (1969) showed that in *Drosophila* methyl- and phenylmercury hydroxides interfere with disjunction of chromosomes in mitosis, and induce recessive sex-linked lethal and visible mutations (in a Muller-5 test). In man, clastogenic effects were shown in *in vitro* cultured lymphocytes (Fiskesjö, 1970).

In Japan, chromosomal lesions were detected several times in blood cells of persons used to eating rather large quantities of raw fish according to the custom of the country (Moriyama, 1968). This observation was confirmed in

Sweden (Skerfving *et al.*, 1970). In this country, the sale of fish containing more than 1 mg per kg (1 ppm of mercury) was prohibited in 1967, and the health authorities warned the population that some fish could originate from polluted areas. Organomercury compounds not only occur preferentially in fish but also in the environment itself and in various conditions: e.g. other foods (from added pesticides), combustion gases, pesticides. Only twelve pesticides among 317 contain mercury, but they are among the most widely utilized. Epstein and Legator (1971, in Gen. Refs.) pointed out that, in the United States, more than 400 000 kg of mercury (15% of the annual production) are used to prepare insecticides.

A certain amount of mercurial residues can persist for years in polluted lakes. This raises alarming problems. What is the average daily exposure of a man to these mercurial molecules? An exact estimation is of course almost impossible.

On the way to his place of work or sometimes at work itself, a worker can inhale a certain quantity of such substance (e.g. methylmercury hydroxide has been identified in combustion gases).

In a meal, a few ppm can be ingested depending on the food, e.g. some fish (see above; Norén and Westöö, 1967; Westöö, 1967) or some plant species in which they accumulate after repeated spraying with pesticides. Fortunately, the whole amount of mercury possibly contained in a food will not be in a mutagenic form. Consequently, measurement of the quantity of mercury in food or even in a more general way in the whole environment is not sufficient to assess the mutagenic risks; it would probably be an overestimation. Mainly organic molecules like methyl- or phenylmercury hydroxide have to be taken into account. If to the absorption of a daily dose, we add inhalation and ingestion of pollutants, cutaneous uptake or even injections of pharmaceuticals containing organomercury compounds, the accumulation in the gonads is such that it will probably reach the critical threshold for mutagenicity.

The metabolism of organomercury derivatives was carefully investigated in man (Åberg *et al.*, 1969). There are indications that some derivatives thought to be inocuous can participate in mutagenic biosyntheses under specific conditions (Jensen and Jernelöv, 1969). In this case, they should be considered, rather as hidden mutagens (Chapter 7).

The genetic risks of organometallic derivatives are far from being limited to organomercury compounds. Other heavy metals occur in numerous places. They are found as impurities in relatively high proportion either in industry or, to a lesser extent, in foods and drugs. They have been investigated for their own potential mutagenicity. It is not improbable that they have synergistic effects between themselves or with other, normally weak, mutagens. The clastogenicity and mutagenicity of heavy metals and derivatives have been reviewed: for arsenic see Léonard and Lauwerys (1980a); for lead see Gerber *et al.* (1980); for chromium, Léonard and Lauwerys (1980b); for cadmium, Degraeve (1981); and for nickel, Léonard *et al.* (1981). Some arsenic derivatives are considered powerful clastogens in mammalian cells, and induce a significant increase of crossing-over frequency in *Drosophila*. The mutagenicity of these arsenic derivatives in a dominant lethal assay in mouse has to be demonstrated.

Organic arsenicals are known to change considerably the spectrum of genetic effects induced by the alkylating agent ethylmethane sulphonate (Moutschen *et al.*, 1965). The cases of lead and nickel derivatives are less disturbing. Lead is known to concentrate in cell nuclei. At high doses it can show cytotoxicity, but its mutagenicity is still questionable. As for nickel, the relatively small number of studies on its derivatives does not allow one to conclude that it is actually mutagenic. Chromium too does not seem to be highly mutagenic, but some derivatives induce chromosome damage and increase the frequency of sister-chromatid exchanges in cultures of mammalian cells. A quite important genetic effect has been described. These derivatives arrest spermatogenesis in rat, and can result in temporary sterility. Clastogenic effects of cadmium were described in plants, but it has only weak effects in mammalian cells *in vivo* or *in vitro* at high doses. The sex-linked recessive lethal test in *Drosophila* and dominant lethal mutation assay in mouse gave negative results. However, in mammals, some doses induced an irreversible testicular atrophy. In experiments on human lymphocytes treated with lead, cadmium and zinc acetates, alone or in combinations of two of the salts, or the three together, only chromosomes treated with solutions containing cadmium showed chromosome damage (Gasiorek and Bauchinger, 1981). This experiment, and others of the same type, are interesting models since humans, particularly workers in factories, are exposed to multiple hazards in conditions such that effects are cumulated.

Two additional points should be mentioned concerning the potential hazards of heavy metals:

(1) As stated above for arsenicals, they can interact with molecules of quite remote classes, possibly at quite different levels, i.e. in the environment or in the human body.

(2) The most important risk of such compounds is probably the risk of carcinogenicity which should be taken into account urgently.

There are many examples of substances found in such conditions to which man is inevitably exposed more than once a day, and in such a way that the effects of the first exposure would not have time to disappear before the second exposure. In all cases where detoxification processes are overloaded, the substance can concentrate in the gonads and then show its mutagenic effects. This stresses once more the importance of information on the 'gonad-dose'. To define this dose, the concentration of the substance actually measured in these organs should be known. Fortunately, natural histological barriers modify and generally decrease diffusion into the gonads of a variety of substances. Moreover, the gonads have also to some extent the capacity to detoxify various subtances, thus decreasing or preventing genetic effects.

The interaction of cofactors is well known in mutagenesis. Several researchers showed the possibility of changing considerably the mutation spectra of some alkylating agents by adding quantities, sometimes extraordinarily low amounts, of substances such as copper or zinc salts or arsenicals commonly found as impurities in the environment (Moutschen and Moutschen-Dahmen, 1963a, b; Moutschen, 1965; Moutschen *et al.*, 1965; Bari, 1963; Bhatia and Narajanan, 1965; Gilot *et al.*, 1967). Fig. 36 shows the effects of salts on different kinds of mutation induced by ethyl methanesulphonate. This substance, known to be one of the most efficient mutagens, is fortunately not used much, except sometimes in the photographic industry.

The principle of comutagenic activity has now been generally adopted in experimental mutagenesis, and it is to be expected that in daily life one will find in the environment numerous 'cofactors' potentiating mutagenic substances more frequently than antagonizing them. In Chapter 4, we said that after a long controversy caffeine was not considered to induce mutagenic effects in mammals (survey in Timson, 1977). There is, however, one more complex view of this question.

Table 7 summarizes some results of selected research performed along different lines. Some agents, e.g. UV light, have been investigated in detail.

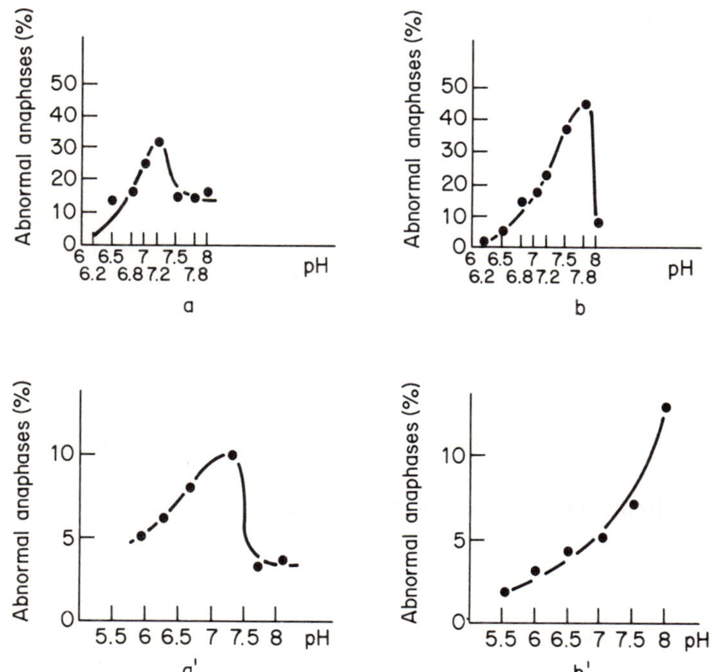

FIG. 36. Modifications by various 'cofactors' of the effects of a sulphonate (ethyl methanesulphonate, EMS) on broad bean seeds (a and b) and barley caryopses (a′ and b′). a: zinc sulphate; b: copper sulphate; a′: mercury dishloride; b′: neo-arsphenamine (arsenic derivative).
In these experimental conditions, control (EMS without 'cofactor') shows few clastogenic effects. Interaction between comutagen and mutagen is strongly pH dependent. (a and b: from Moutschen *et al.*, 1965); a′ and b′: from Moutschen and Moutschen-Dahmen, 2963.)

TABLE 7. Modifications by cofactors of the mutagenic action of caffeine, (review in Adler in Röhrborn and Vogel, 1970, and Timson, 1977)

Author	Experimental material	Cofactor	Effect
Witkin (1958)	Bacteria	UV	Synergistic
		Purinenucleotides	Antagonist
Lieb (1961)	Bacteria	UV	Synergistic
Rauth (1967)	Mouse cultured cells	UV	Synergistic
Jacobson (in Kuhlman *et al.* (1968)	Human leucocytes	X-rays	Synergistic
Wragg *et al.* (1967)	Human leucocytes	Mitomycin C	Synergistic
Hixon and Yielding (1976)	Yeast	Ethidium bromide	Antagonist
Brøgger (1974)	Human lymphocytes	Methyl methane sulphonate	Synergistic
Nemirovskii and Klimenko (1973)	Rat hepatocytes	Dipine (alkylating agent)	Antagonist

They do not seem to result in practical applications, but it is not excluded that common compounds such as ethyl alcohol or Versene (a food additive mentioned in Chapter 4) might have synergistic effects with caffeine.

The fact that the list of potential 'cofactors' is growing fast should be emphasized. Apart from fortuitous 'cofactors', interactions between substances belonging to remote chemical classes are by far the most frequent. The number of interactions demonstrated is rapidly increasing and does not grow proportionally to man's wisdom.

Another field where comutagenicity has been investigated is that of cooked food. The relatively recent finding of potential mutagenicity in some cooked foods pointed out the urgent need to investigate this problem as a whole (see also Chapter 4). Two comutagenic substances were isolated from the tar of tryptophan pyrolysates, namely harman and norharman. The pyrolysates extracted from cooked meat (Trp-P-1 and Trp-P-2) showed enhanced mutagenic activity in the presence of harman and norharman in *Salmonella typhimurium* TA98. This enhancement requires activation by microsomal enzymes (review in Tazima, 1982). The mechanism of comutagenic action has not yet been elucidated, but there are good reasons to think that the two comutagenic substances intercalate in the DNA molecule. This underlines the fact that intercalating substances which by themselves show weak mutagenicity could enhance or even determine the effects of unrelated substances.

In bacteria, the mutagenic activity of benzo(*a*)pyrene, a well known carcinogenic substance in mammals, was also enhanced by harman and norharman

(Nagao *et al.*, 1975, quoted in Tazima, 1982). It is likely that synergistic effects are also produced with other carcinogenic substances requiring activation. The comutagenic effect of norharman was also described with aminopyrene (Wakabayashi *et al.*, 1982), which belongs to a completely different group of substances. This synergism does not seem to occur in man, possibly due to metabolic differences.

The above-mentioned reactions are far from being the only ones that occur in such complex media as foods. Kada (1973) obtained mutagenic substances by mixing two additives: the harmless sorbic acid with the less harmless sodium nitrite (mutagenicity described in Chapter 7). Hayato and his coworkers (quoted in Tazima, 1982) isolated three mutagenic substances. Two of them have been identified (Hartman, 1983). The formation of the mutagenic substances is in this case clearly in the environment, i.e. in the food before entering the cell.

The question of the mutagenicity of foodstuffs is highly complex. In fact, foods are also known to contain substances which transform mutagens already existing or just formed into non-mutagenic substances (desmutagens), or alternatively which antagonize the mutagenic action in the body (antimutagens). Examples of these substances will be given in Chapter 10. It can be concluded from this research, and in view of the complexity and the diversity of the problems, that the control of foodstuffs should certainly be reinforced by adequate genetic tests. But in this field, maybe more than in others, the choice of the right battery of tests will be difficult, but certainly not more difficult than changing the feeding habits of individuals.

Interaction mechanisms between two or more substances are numerous. In the previous chapter, we noted examples in which non-mutagenic and even non-toxic compounds become active by chemical reactions, *inter se* either in the environment or in the human body, and sometimes in both successively. The interactions to which we allude in the present chapter do not involve, except when otherwise stated, chemical reactions between two or more substances resulting in a mutagenic combination. So it is demonstrated that DDT and related substances or other chlorinated hydrocarbons accumulate in fats of living beings. Although we reported in Chapter 4, the clastogenic and mutagenic potential of several pesticides, their concentration in the gonads is often not high enough to induce an effect. However, even in such conditions, it is well established that these molecules considerably stimulate the production of microsomal liver enzymes. Following such stimulation the metabolism of a variety of substances is strongly enhanced. This is advantageous in most cases, but when metabolic transformations activate mutagenic properties such enhanced metabolism allows the critical threshold to be quickly reached (review in de Serres *et al.*, 1976, in Gen. Refs., and Scott *et al.*, 1977, in Gen. Refs.)

Table 8 indicates that concentrations of various insecticides measured in the human body are sufficiently high to provoke interactions. In rat, a single intraperitoneal injection of even a very small quantity of DDT can activate the metabolism of several substances, including barbiturates, for periods as long as

Table 8. Some examples of pesticides found in peritoneal fat of inhabitants of four American cities (modified from Zavon, 1969)

Pesticides	Men (41 cases) Mean ppm	Women (23 cases) Mean ppm	Total (64 cases) Mean ppm
Dieldrin*	0.31	0.24	0.28
DDE	5.39	3.61	4.75
o,p-DDT	0.21	0.11	0.17
p,p-DDT	2.52	2.18	2.40
Heptachloride epoxide	0.11	0.09	0.10

* 1, 2, 3, 4, 10–Hexachloro-6, 7-epoxi-1, 4, 4a, 5, 6, 7, 8, 8a-octahydro-1, 4-*endo-exo*-5, 8-dimethanonaphthalene

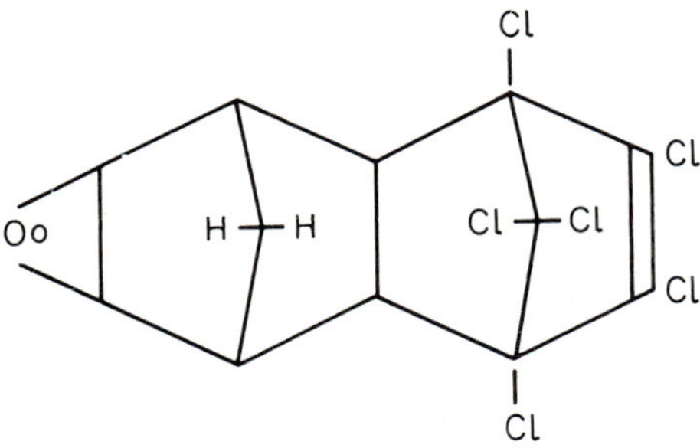

60–90 days (Ghazal *et al.*, 1964; Conney, 1967).

McLean (1965) showed that the exaggerated production of liver microsomal enzymes can transform a compound such as (2-acetylaminofluorene) into an efficient carcinogen. Transformations leading to synergistic actions can also occur not only with the numerous pesticides flooding the market, but also with food additives, pharmaceuticals, and air and water pollutants. These synergistic effects should be carefully checked and investigated in detail. One difficulty lies in the fact that, in this field, animal experiments are relatively less efficient due to the differences between mammalian and human metabolism. Tests of metabolic control of mutagens in man should be developed (e.g. in blood, urine and amniotic fluid: see Chapter 9) in all cases where there is reason to suppose that interactions can occur.

During the last few years, a great effort has been made to identify potentially hazardous ambient air pollutants, and also potentially mutagenic substances in water, especially drinking water. There are various ways to proceed. The first approach is to collect samples from all polluted areas (industrial or otherwise) where mutagenic or carcinogenic compounds are suspected to occur. The second step is to isolate fractions by chemical techniques, and to test them separately using suitable test systems.

When a mutagenic substance is detected, it needs to be identified at the molecular level. This is far from being a routine test! The detection of all possible interactions either synergistic or antagonistic will be the final and crucial step of this long journey. The second approach to identifying environmental hazards complements the first. It is not so analytical but, at the present stage, may be more rewarding. The method is to place bio-indicators of genotoxicity wherever a hazard is suspected, as a kind of biological dosimeter. Such assays have the merit of indicating at least what and where the problems are. For ambient air pollutants, some important guidelines for future investigations have emerged (Hughes *et al.*, 1980; Chrisp and Fisher, 1980; Whong *et al.*, 1981). The analytical approach first suggested is to separate two phases — the vapour phase and the particulate phase — by chemical extractions, because these phases have different genetic implications. The methodology for each phase follows different procedures.

The sources of contamination are quite diverse; for example, automobile and diesel exhaust, coal fly ash, welding fumes, cigarette smoke. Some environmental factors are critical such as UV irradiation, wind and humidity.

It is not surprising that, in such conditions, many interactions occur with potential cumulative effects. These interactions are far from being equally investigated. Diesel fuel has received particular attention. An interaction was found between diesel fuel and nitrite which produces a direct mutagen for bacteria without needing activation by microsomal fractions (Henderson *et al.*, 1981). Most of the isolated fractions were tested on bacteria, in an Ames test, except cigarette smoke which deserved more extensive studies. In fact, cigarette smoke condensate was found to be mutagenic in a variety of test systems: *Salmonella typhimurium* and *Neurospora crassa* (Demarini, 1981a, b), sex-linked recessive lethal mutations in *Drosophila melanogaster* (Pescitelli, 1979), increased sister-chromatid exchanges in Chinese hamster ovary cells, and in the Ames test (De Raat, 1979). From these abundant data, it can certainly be concluded that cigarette smoke is a real genetic hazard, besides the well-known carcinogenic effect. But how are we going to change the life-style of people? The strategies for identifying the priorities in pollution research are sometimes ill-defined, and new models should be continually worked out. An attractive model, recently developed, is based on the knowledge of organ-specific toxicity. For example, for air-borne particles, the smallest particles have been found to show the highest mutagenicity in the Ames test. Keeping in mind the affinity of these particles for lung tissue, it becomes obvious that this fraction deserves special detailed investigations. Along the same line, experiments were designed to investigate the extractive properties of physiological body fluids (King *et al.*, 1981). They were found to differ greatly from the solvents commonly used for separating the fraction that contains the smallest particles. It could be demonstrated that the mutagenicity of diesel particle organics is greatly reduced by the addition of serum or of lung cytosol (King *et al.*, 1981). Such assays should certainly be fostered, since in this specific field the results can be of help in cancer prophylaxis. The problems of interaction are surely no less easy to solve in complex aqueous media, especially drinking water (review in Loper, 1980). In this latter case, important problems have been identified. The first is that water contains volatile compounds, which involves a special methodology for mutagenicity testing. Another problem is that the components of water and therefore their potential mutagenicity are quite variable with the season, depending especially on disinfection which is generally made by chlorination. This has at least two consequences. The first is that tests should be repeatedly performed. The second is that an adequate battery of tests should be selected according to the season. Almost all the tests for mutagenicity of drinking water have been performed with bacteria, which are certainly not the best organisms to use when disinfectants are present! In the field of air and water pollution, the gate for future research into mutagenic and comutagenic substances is still wide open.

Concerning the second approach to control of the environment, several biological indicators of pollution have long been recommended in classical toxicology, e.g. lichens, which are particularly sensitive to toxic substances. Long ago the World Health Organization surveyed the problem (WHO, 1963). Unfortunately, these bio-indicators of pollution have poor specificity, and provide little information on genetic effects. This is the reason why new bio-indicators of mutagenic substances should be developed.

The traditional *Tradescantia* pollen test (Chapter 2) has been recommended and successfully applied to the solution of environmental problems (Schairer *et al.*, 1978a, b; Van't Hof and Schairer, 1982) at specific industrial sites. The effects of effluents from a lead smelting plant were also investigated using the same test system (Lower *et al.*, 1978). Other bio-indicator plant species were also proposed, such as maize (Plewa and Gentile, 1976) and soybean (quoted in Hughes *et al.*, 1980).* An attractive idea was proposed and has already been applied in specific programmes. This is to use a movable laboratory which not only performs short-term experiments with bio-indicators, but equally is equipped to detect or even identify chemical contaminants.

* Some bio-indicators are briefly described in Chapter 3 (some reflections). Problems of control of the environment will also be discussed in Chapter 9.

Chapter 9

The Necessity for Considering the Environment as a Whole

'Denn nicht durch den Besitz, sondern durch die Forschung nach Wahrheit erweitern sich seine Kräfte, worin allein seine immer wachsende Vollkomenheit besteht'

Lessing
(*Minna von Barnhelm*)

In Chapter 4, we looked for all possible sources of potential mutagens in the environment. For several reasons, some agents are difficult to detect, and some substances normally innocuous *in vitro* can require mutagenicity after reactions *in vivo* (Chapter 7).

Methods of detection have been briefly described in Chapters 1 and 2. Some of these methods, even when they are not sufficiently elaborate, allow one to conclude that widespread mutagenic agents generate multiple genetic risks, especially because of the possibility of cumulative effects and interactions (Chapter 8).

These considerations strongly indicate that the mutagenicity of the environment should be considered as a whole instead of identifying each problem separately and of analysing the effects under specific laboratory conditions as we did previously. The risks will be more accurately assessed if the problem is analysed in its entire complexity.

ACCUMULATION OF MUTAGENIC SUBSTANCES AND AMPLIFICATION OF EFFECTS IN THE TROPHIC CHAIN

A first problem, alarming for man in the short term, results from the fact that many contaminants are not directly biodegradable but enter the trophic chain in which they can accumulate in a sometimes unforeseeable way. This accumulative process which results in amplified effects can be illustrated by examples of numerous pollutants, the mutagenic effects of which have been separately and repeatedly investigated in laboratories. In this context, radioactive compounds are surely the best example to describe first. When waste containing radioactive compounds with long half-lives is incidentally or accidentally discharged into an aqueous medium such as a river or a lake, components of the phytoplankton such as algae and bacteria rapidly fix a significant part of the radioactivity. Foster and Rostenbach (1954) measured in

Columbia river phytoplankton an accumulation of radiophosphorus one thousand times that of the background.

This concentration of radioactive wastes occurs not only in fresh water phytoplankton but also in marine phytoplankton. At this early stage the accumulation of radioactive matter is already a hazard if we keep in mind that diverse species of algae can be used by man, e.g. as food. But this phytoplankton will in turn be eaten by aquatic insects which continue the concentration process without too much damage to themselves since these organisms are generally very insensitive to radiation. This accumulation of radioactivity in the trophic chain will continue in mollusc, crustacea, and particularly fish. At the end of the amplification processes the genetic risks will become quite impressive if we remember the powerful mutagenic effects of ionizing radiations (Chapter 6). Radioactive compounds can be scattered sometimes at very long distances from the source of the pollution, especially by migratory birds. Moreover, radioactive contaminants can arise from multiple origins, not only from nuclear industries but also from chance contaminations and radioactive fall-out. This classical example of accumulation of radioactive contaminants by the trophic chain is sufficient to show that the exact evaluation of genetic hazards of ionizing radiations should first be based on knowledge of the movement of radioactive matter through the whole biosphere.

The general process of accumulation of radioactive waste can be extended to a large number of contaminants. We are already familiar with the effects of pesticides (Chapters 4, 5 and 7). Corn is often sprayed with insecticides, including dieldrin. The spraying is usually extensive and repeated, excess quantities being intended to protract the effects. In Great Britain, it was found that a rather large number of granivorous birds such as ring-doves died unexpectedly. It was gradually established that this process extended to predatory birds such as eagles and falcons, and even to mammals such as foxes. An investigation revealed that this effect could only occur through their prey. This was confirmed by further investigations showing that the chemically stable dieldrin accumulates in granivorous birds, and reaches a lethal level. It has further been demonstrated that dieldrin has mutagenic properties at doses much lower than those at which the first toxic effects are observed (Markarian, 1967). This is far from being a unique example of toxic accumulation in the trophic chain!

Among the genetic hazards of pesticides mutagenic effects are often mentioned, but it is now evident that the effects on selective and recombinational processes should also be investigated. The consequences of such modifications are at present impossible to foresee and, probably, to avoid.

It can certainly be concluded that permanent risks for man are far beyond those of a single chance contamination by just one pollutant.

Although the accumulation in the trophic chain of substances capable of deleterious effects on man is a matter for concern, the trophic chain can inversely screen off many poisons. Plants too have efficient detoxification mechanisms active for numerous mutagenic compounds. Without such detoxification mechanisms, many compounds would reach man in far higher concentrations. This is, for instance, the case for gaseous compounds at room temperature, such as the ubiquitous ethylene oxide, nitrosamines and some aldehydes (described in Chapters 4, 5 and 7). The role played by plants in detoxifying mutagenic substances is but a particular case of fixation of the most varied noxious substances appearing in the biosphere. This stresses the need to maintain or even to develop 'green areas', especially around cities.

ENVIRONMENTAL MUTAGENS: BLIND EVOLUTIVE FACTORS

Another point worth surveying in the field of environmental mutagenesis is that mutagenic agents not only concern man but, in fact, all living beings.

It has been demonstrated that in the present conditions of use they can act as powerful, generally uncontrolled, evolutive factors. The fact that mutagenic effects are far from being the only ones resulting in genetic modifications of populations has already been stressed. According to Stebbins (1957, in Gen. Refs., 1959), and this is still the opinion of numerous researchers, the evolution of higher animals and plants depends on four distinct processes: mutations, genetic recombination, natural selection and isolating mechanisms of populations. Numerous agents, especially pesticides, can act simultaneously or successively at these four levels.

In 1972, Gustafsson wrote: 'Pesticide chemicals, originally used to help mankind survive, do not only destroy injurious elements of life, they also harm the balanced interaction of the system and the entirety itself.'

The dumping of large amounts of pesticides in the environment has multiple consequences, and the different facets of the problem can scarcely be separated.

Already in 1931, Kostoff described chromosomal lesions in cells of tobacco plants, the seeds of which had been submitted to fumigation with nicotine sulphate. Numerous meiotic anomalies were observed, resulting in almost complete sterility. Substances such as carbamates are components of a whole class of pesticides. Marked polyploidizing effects of such compounds were reported (Mann and Storey, 1966). Several animal feeds, e.g. alfalfa (luzern), and sunflower seem particularly sensitive to this kind of agent (Van den Born, 1969). Several mutants, sometimes major, were observed even a long time after the removal of the pesticide from the soil. Grant (1972) studied the mutagenic effects of pesticides in detail. Naming them 'subtle promoters of evolution' he observed all kinds of chromosomal effects which can be induced by the most powerful mutagens (e.g. alkylating agents) after treatment of barley root tips.

In Fig. 37 the effects of some pesticides are compared with the effects of an X-ray dose giving 50% sterility in barley (Grant, 1970). These examples show the mutagenic efficiency of pesticides in plants. As far as animals are concerned, the effects are possibly of much less significance though some lesions have been repeatedly described in insects, especially *Drosophila*, and even in mammals.

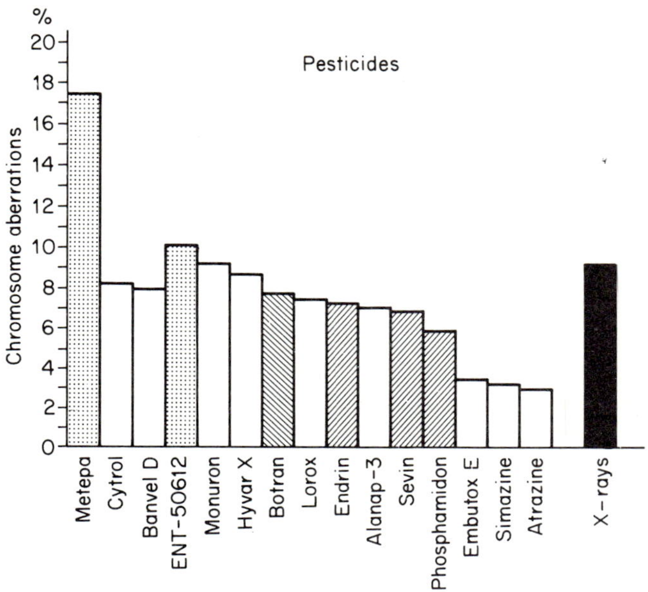

FIG. 37. Comparison between the effects of X-rays (5000 R) and various pesticides on *Vicia faba* root tips (pesticide concentration in aqueous solution is near saturation). (After Grant, 1970.)

Another peculiar mechanism by which pesticides can act as evolutive (or rather involutive!) factors on animal and plant species, independently from their mutagenic potential, is by selection pressure which is the consequence of indiscriminate killing of the species or varieties. In fact, artificial selection, when replacing natural selection, after abuse of pesticides can lead to unpredicted consequences at the population level. First, the blind destruction of sensitive species or varieties favours the proliferation of other organisms sometimes more undesirable than those that were supposed to be eradicated. Such examples of breakdown of natural equilibria are numerous, and have been abundantly described in plants. In the plant kingdom, especially, an unexpected consequence of such breakdown would be the complete extinction of wild stocks which still have an important role to play in the improvement of domestic species.

In fact, among these wild species, we can find the ancestry of our cultivated species; this is especially so for cereals (e.g. wheat, maize, rice).

Famous works of Vavilov (published in 1949–1950, in Gen. Refs.) pertinently showed the major interest in tracing back the ancestry of our cultivated species. It would allow cultivated specimens to be back-crossed with these selected ancestors for conferring desirable characters on hybrid species, thereby managing a reserve of variability and adaptability. This is still a classical method of improving plant species. In this way it would be possible to create varieties resistant to adverse conditions.

The survival of a species depends upon its potential of variability. If this variability is depleted too much, it is to be expected that many cultivated varieties which are among the best successes of plant growers will be annihilated by slight changes of environment such as new pathogenic germs, a hard winter or too dry a summer (review in Frankel and Bennett, 1970, in Gen. Refs.)

Are excessive sprayings with pesticides going to deprive man of one of the most efficient methods of improving plant species or ruin centuries of constant endeavour?

We have less information concerning the two last processes through which pesticides could act as evolutive factors. On the one hand, it is clear to the population geneticists that the irreversible disappearance of a species from a sufficiently large geographical area will generally result in the isolation of other species. This isolation is another powerful evolutive factor. On the other hand, the effects of pesticides on recombination are almost completely unknown. Since they are obviously important evolutive mechanisms, it would be desirable to investigate such effects. We should once more emphasize the difficulty of dissociating all these effects at the population level, whether mutagenic, selective or recombinogenic. Extrapolation of the hazards to man should take all these factors into account.

Another important chapter of genetic toxicology derived from the preceding considerations is the control of human populations themselves.

SURVEILLANCE AND MONITORING OF HUMAN POPULATIONS

Surveillance of human populations can be performed at two levels, in some ways complementary. The first is the surveillance of the population itself, and the second is the control of the environment where the population is living. The question is: Which populations should be checked? The answer is: first those populations with the highest occupational hazards. The requirements for occupational surveillance of workers differ greatly from one industry to another, and even within the same industry. The controls should obviously be more frequent for workers continuously submitted to dangerous agents such as, for example, in the rubber and petroleum industries, ionizing radiations, and in industries producing vinyl chloride. These epidemiological studies are made difficult for many reasons mainly due to the diversity of the populations investigated and the large number of parameters involved. The nature of the genotoxic contaminants is infrequently known exactly. They are generally complex mixtures not only involving a main substance such as the familiar 'environmental mobsters' vinyl chloride or ethylene oxide, but also potentially genotoxic impurities occurring sometimes in high concentrations. The analysis of the effects of complex mixtures requires special methodology. First, as stated in Chapters 7 and 8 in which examples are given, components can react together giving rise to a mutagenic compound. Second, when the mixture contains highly toxic substances they mask other less toxic but highly mutagenetic substances. The dose of genotoxic mixtures absorbed is another badly known variable, depending on things like the place of work, the degree of pollution which changes from time to time according to the method of manufacture and also the workers' conditions, in particular the means of protection. At the present stage of progress in epidemiological studies, the solutions proposed for surveillance of populations are still empirical. After identifying the population to be regularly examined, what controls should be done? In this matter, there are two distinct but complementary approaches. The first is cytogenetic surveillance, which attempts to evaluate chromosomal damage in lymphocytes of workers (review in Kilian and Picciano, 1976). The second is the analysis of the body fluids, which aims to detect mutagenic metabolites (review in Legator *et al.*, 1978). The techniques available to prepare cells for clastogenic analysis are quite simple (details in Chapter 2). A blood sample is taken and enriched in lymphocytes in which mitoses are initiated by adding phytohaemagglutinin extracted from kidney beans. After adding colchicine to the sample for increasing the number of metaphases, slides are prepared for analysis of chromosomal damage. Then the problems arise! First, this analysis is far from being routine work. It demands long professional training, and it is time-consuming. For the sake of simplicity and saving time, analysis of the damage is often limited to the most evident aberrations: dicentric chromosomes (examples in Fig. 7, Chapter 2). This is quite a biased estimation of the real damage. It has also been suggested to score sister-chromatid exchanges as an alternative to chromosome breakage. This could more easily become a routine technique, with the disadvantages mentioned in Chapter 3. Besides the above-mentioned limitations of the cytogenetic surveillance, another difficulty arises from the extreme heterogeneity of the human populations investigated, not only due to differences of exposure to various agents, but also to differences of genetic background, life-style and even chance factors. The population submitted to occupational surveillance should be examined at regular intervals, the frequency of which depends on the levels of contamination. This population should also be compared with a control population, not submitted to the same hazards. The appropriate choice of this reference population is difficult. It is clear that a large proportion of lymphocyte donors should be avoided, including persons who were recently exposed to well-known mutagens, persons suffering from diseases in which high frequencies of chromosomal aberrations occur such as Fanconi's anaemia, Bloom's syndrome, ataxia telangiectasia, xeroderma pigmentosum, persons suffering from infections especially virus, and finally the many heavy smokers and drug addicts. Since the ideal control will not be easy to find, the level of clastogenicity in the reference population has to be established on average. Sperm has also been suggested for surveillance of workers. (David *et al.*, 1975). An interesting possibility is the staining of the so-called F-bodies with fluorescent probes. This allows non-disjunction of Y chromosomes to be detected (e.g. Kapp and Jacobson, 1980) using the Beatty technique (Beatty, 1977; see Chapter 2).

More recent techniques (described in Chapter 2) for scoring somatic biochemical mutant cells are rapidly developing. When automated, they will certainly be applicable to population surveillance and monitoring. They will efficiently complement chromosome damage analysis.

The second possibility for population surveillance and monitoring is the examination of body fluids. There are several ways to look at the problem. Urine fractions in which it is reasonable to suspect mutagenic potential can be tested after separating different components. The rapid screening tests have the disadvantages reported in Chapter 3 for lower organisms. In fact, various test systems have actually been utilized. *Salmonella typhimurium* was used in an Ames test (Durston and Ames, 1974). Siebert (1973) worked out a technique based on the induction of prototrophic mutants from a defective yeast strain, and on a genic conversion of heteroallelic loci. Using this test system, Siebert (1973) and Siebert and Simon (1973a, b) demonstrated the mutagenic properties of the urine (and amniotic fluid) of a patient treated with cyclophosphamide (Cytosan, Endoxan). This promutagen is known to be converted to a mutagen (Fig. 11, Chapter 2). Cultured human lymphocytes were also tested (Chebotarer *et al.*, 1976) and whole organisms such as *Drosophila* (Browing, 1973). Body fluids other than urine, namely blood, amniotic fluid and sperm, are also used for population monitoring. Blood is at least as important as urine for detecting potentially mutagenic metabolites which might accumulate in the circulatory system, and eventually cross the gonad barrier. Blood has also been recommended for the detection of reactions with macromolecules, DNA or proteins by the techniques briefly described in Chapter 1. These are generally alkylation reactions of great importance. For example, in mouse the reactivity of tissue proteins for monofunctional alkylating agents such as ethylene oxide is 1.5 to 5 times higher than for DNA (Ehrenberg *et al.,* 1974). For technical reasons haemoglobin is generally preferred to DNA. A blood sample of only 10–20 ml is required for a complete investigation. Standard methods of isolating alkylated amino acids from haemoglobin were used to develop a test of very high resolving power (Osterman-Golkar *et al.*, 1976, 1977; Segerbäck *et al.*, 1978). It was shown that several amino acids are alkylated, principally cysteine, histidine, methionine and serine, but histidine is the most convenient for quantitative analysis. Thanks to the possibility of using radiolabelled monofunctional alkylating agents, the power of resolution for detecting risks was estimated to be 10^{-4} rad-equivalents (definition in Chapter 10) (Ehrenberg and Osterman-Golkar, 1980). Since the lifespan of red blood cells is of the order of 125 days in man, surveillance can be carried out for a long time.

Another interesting source of information is bile. It hardly needs mentioning that several compounds belonging to various chemical classes are substantially excreted into the bile. Properties of detoxification or alternatively activation into mutagens have been described. Thus bile as a body fluid can be used in test systems for *in vitro* studies of, for example, liver microsomal fractions or for *in vivo* studies. For obvious reasons, investigations on bile can only be carried out in animals. Good experimental data are quite valuable for understanding the role of this body fluid in metabolically changing the mutagenicity of compounds. Therefore such data are relevant for population monitoring.

Salmonella typhimurium was used first as a test system to investigate the detoxifying properties of bile (Rannug and Beije, 1978; Connor *et al.*, 1979). Attention was drawn to the fact that aromatic amines are particularly excreted into the bile either as non-mutagenic glucuronate conjugates or as mutagenic metabolites of the compound (Connor *et al.*, 1979).

In the context of occupational surveillance, it is also important to investigate faeces. In some circumstances, enteric bacteria are known to convert promutagens into mutagens. This has occasionally been demonstrated for drugs (review in Scheline, 1973). Kuhnlein *et al.* (1981) detected faecal mutagens in a fluctuation test on *Salmonella typhimurium* designed to identify weak mutagens. They separated two active substances, and made the peculiar observation that vegetarians have significantly lower levels of such mutagens. At least such research could help monitor dietary programmes!

The risks of substances taken orally, e.g. drugs, will certainly be greater than the risks of substances taken by other routes. However, it is not ruled out that such risks of enteric activation do not exist after exposure to substances absorbed by another route as in industrial pollution.

In view of the above examples, it is clear that faeces should also be controlled for mutagenicity. Since such controls can not be routinely performed on a large scale, the decision for surveillance will finally be based on knowledge of the substances to which workers are exposed, and, of course, on metabolic studies of these substances.

During the last decade, efforts were made to correlate carcinogenicity and mutagenicity by evaluating the information obtained in short-term tests (review in Clayson, 1980). The rationale for establishing a correlation is as follows. To become effective either as a mutagen or a carcinogen, many substances should first be transformed into electrophiles, i.e. compounds reacting strongly with important targets such as DNA, RNA and proteins. These transformations occur *in vivo,* and to a lesser extent *in vitro*. Therefore, if substances capable of inducing cancers in mammals are proved to be transformed *in vitro* into genotoxic compounds after addition of microsomal fractions, the correlation is sustained. For example, benzo(*a*)pyrene, a well-known carcinogen, is converted into a strong mutagen by adding mouse liver microsomes to the medium of treated bacteria (*Salmonella*) (Oesch *et al.*, 1976, 1977). In spite of numerous experiments, carcinogenic hydrocarbons from coal-tar show quite a low mutagenicity in mammals (Strong, 1948). Differences in metabolic pathways between mammalian cells and bacteria often lead to misinterpretations of the results. On the one hand, if bacteria detoxify the compound under test, whereas mammalian tissues are unable to do so, the test does not detect any mutagenic effect, whether or not the microsomal fraction is added. This is a *false negative* result.

On the other hand, if mammalian cells detoxify the compound but the bacteria do not, then the bacterial test will show mutagenicity. This is a *false positive*. Normally, the mutagenic effect should disappear when microsomal fractions are added. Being of mammalian origin these fractions should contain the whole enzymatic equipment needed for detoxification. However, it should be remembered that the addition of microsomal fractions *in vitro* is only a very approximate model of what happens *in vivo*. Such fractions mimic very incompletely the *in vivo* metabolic pathways, ignoring quite important things such as the route of administration of the compound, its distribution in the body, its excretion and also tissue specificities of enzymes.

If the correlation is demonstrated in a large majority of cases, it seems possible to use short-term tests systematically as indicators of potential carcinogenicity before performing long-term experiments of cancer induction in mammals.

Now, how good are the above correlations and how valid are such methods? It was stated that the Ames test with *Salmonella typhimurium* agrees in 80–90% of the cases with long-term bioassays (Ames *et al.*, 1977). What about the 10–20% of remaining substances for which there are discrepancies between the results of short-term tests and long-term bioassays? The reasons for such discrepancies are not yet clear. There are some possible explanations, however. First, the test is not adequate for various substances and also in various conditions. Substances such as metals, chlorocarbon carcinogens, some hormones, cannot be tested by these procedures. Other substances known to participate actively in malignancy do not act via genotoxicity but by epigenetic mechanisms modifying growth control (review in Weisburger and Williams, 1982). These substances, which might be more numerous than expected, will of course remain undetected in any genetic test.

Additionally, there are problems in choosing the organ and even the donor organism, and in preparing the microsomal fractions. Often, a positive malignant transformation is obtained with one mammalian species and not with another. Moreover, microsomal fractions prepared from one organ, generally the liver, do not cover the whole field since many malignant tumours are organ- or tissue-specific (review in Schmähl and Pool, 1982). If, for example, lung tissue had been used to prepare the microsomal fractions instead of liver, a genotoxic effect would have been revealed.

Finally, the data from *in vivo* experiments are sometimes difficult to interpret. They are borderline due to too low sample sizes or to the need for highly trained personnel. Are we prepared to accept unreservedly the correlation between carcinogenicity and genotoxicity? Obviously when there are strong positive results in short-term tests, it is an important indication that further tests should be performed (see Chapter 10 for the tests strategy). What about the remaining proportion of negative tests? In such cases the chemical structure of a substance, its metabolic pathways and the importance of its use in human life should serve as guidelines (Wright, 1980)

CONTROL OF THE ENVIRONMENT

It is obvious that some molecules should be limited to definite uses. It is also clear that molecules recently introduced to the environment should be subjected to a battery of relevant tests. Moreover, human populations should be submitted to surveillance and monitoring. Overall control of the environment, however, is still essential.

In this context, it is indispensable to define standards with their confidence limits, bearing in mind that many factors interact to produce genetic effects (Chapter 8). The ambitious project of decontamination of the environment is far beyond the scope of the present problems. It is a problem on a world scale. Decontamination programmes should be organized however, especially in cases where the accidental occurrence or the systematic use of substances raises simultaneously problems of mutagenicity, carcinogenicity and teratogenicity.

Although we emphasized previously the differences of methodology between carcinogenicity and mutagenicity testing, it is true that a large proportion of mutagens are also carcinogens (see above). From this observation, two lines of research have evolved. First, short-term tests for mutagenicity were suggested for testing potential carcinogenic compounds. Conversely, it was suggested to use epidemiological data on cancer occurrences in human populations to predict mutagenicity at further generations. With respect to this second line of research, Ehrenberg (1973) considers that the observation of an increased frequency of cancers and leukaemia in the exposed generation is a biased estimate of mutagenic effects which will only become unmasked in further generations.

There are also agents which, besides carrying a risk of mutagenicity and carcinogenicity disclose a risk of teratogenicity. Such a substance is thalidomide. It showed neither toxic nor genetic effects at doses noxious for the embryos at specific stages. Such substances should be investigated with a particular teratological methodology. Since the respective risks of mutagenicity, carcinogenicity and teratogenicity are somewhat disproportionate in various classes of agents, it would still be wise in spite of the new methodologies cited above to apply the rule of 'limiting factors' the lowest threshold indicating in some ways the methodology to adopt.

Chapter 10

Suggestions for Prophylaxis

'. . . Our stone age genetic constitutions are being sorely stretched in trying to adapt to the unprecedented complications of civilization and of the world as seen by modern science, to the need to feel brotherhood for 3 billion people, and to the responsibility of guiding without disaster the use of the enormous powers that scientific technology has created'

H.J. Muller

(Means and aims in human genetic betterment; in Sonneborn, 1965, in Gen. Refs.)

ESTABLISHING A MODEL

Before making suggestions for prophylaxis, strategies should be defined to test the many potential genetic hazards. Each model for testing is first based on the choice of a reference unit to measure the effects and to assess the risks.

Choice of a reference unit

One of the problems that geneticists tried to solve in the past was to estimate the mutagenic efficiency of a compound by comparing it with the effects of ionizing radiations, taken as a standard. Ehrenberg suggested comparing the genetic effects of alkylating agents with the effects of radiations of low linear energy transfer. This procedure was applied to ethylene oxide; Ehrenberg *et al.* (1974) attempted to define a dose of this substance producing effects comparable to a known dose of radiation. This idea was developed and the name 'rad-equivalent' or *radeq* was proposed for this unit (Bridges, 1973). This procedure is in some ways comparable to the procedure generally adopted for relative biological efficiency, where the effects of one radiation are compared with the well-known effects of another radiation; for example, the effects of neutrons are compared with the effects of X-rays or ^{60}Co or ^{131}Cs γ-rays.

The difficulties of such a procedure are evident:

(1) The mechanisms by which radiations produce their effects are often quite different from those at work for chemicals. They can also differ from one class of substances to another, and even within the same class. Although, it is justified to compare the effects of various ionizing radiations, it is less conceivable to compare chemical agents with physical agents.

(2) The criteria used in genetic toxicology are in general more complex than

those used in classical toxicology, such as survival or growth inhibition. In this context, the estimation of the risks from the analysis of chromosome breakage or alternatively from different classes of point mutations leads to different conclusions. Contrary to ionizing radiations, numerous chemical mutagens induce little or no visible chromosome damage. This is typical, for example, of one nucleoside, nebularine, extracted from mushrooms of the genus *Clitocybe,* which produced a relatively high frequency of point mutations (Ehrenberg *et al.*, 1956) without inducing microscopically visible changes (Moutschen and Moutschen-Dahmen, 1957; quoted in von Wettstein *et al.*, 1959). This is also the case for several purine and pyrimidine analogues; and in specific conditions, and in certain biological systems, it may be the same for ethyl methanesulphonate and even for other alkylating agents. Consequently, the genetic risks of a given dose of a mutagenic chemical can never be exactly equated with the risks of exposure to radiation of the same number of radeqs. It will strictly depend on the criterion chosen unless a considerable number of tests is performed to cover all possible genetics effects.

(3) Contrary to ionizing radiations, some chemicals show a specificity of action such that invariably only one type of lesion is produced. It seems difficult, therefore, to refer to the action of radiations for which the spectrum of mutations is considerably wider. The crucial problem is to know if such extreme specificity found in one organism can also occur in man. It has not been demonstrated. Apart from the limitations indicated above, the choice of the radeq as reference unit should allow the empirical evaluation of the occupational risks of workers exposed to a given substance for long periods, as has been done routinely for workers exposed to radiation in departments of radiology. In this manner, permissible doses could be assessed.

Recently, new concepts have evolved from new experiments in relation to dosimetry. Methods have been developed to analyse the kinetics of mutation induction (Haynes and Eckardt, 1980). Among other things, these methods are based on the concept of relative mutagenic efficiency which takes into account the stochastic dependence of mutation and killing. Let us suppose that two mutagenic agents A and B have the same mutagenic effect at the same selected dose with the same dosimetry and the same criterion of mutagenicity, but that agent B shows higher toxicity than agent A. Because A is less toxic than B, it is expected that more mutants will remain viable. Therefore, a higher dose will be required to reach the maximum yield of mutations. Under specified conditions, relative mutagenic efficiency can be defined as the ratio of the maximum yields of mutations, allowing, in principle, a more direct comparison between the efficiency of two mutagenic agents. The assessment of the ratio will strongly depend on the kinetic patterns of the agents, i.e. the shape of the curves showing dose–effect relations. Knowledge of the kinetic patterns presupposes that a sufficient amount of data can be collected. In practice, this is far from being possible. If so, it is empirically reasonable to assume that, if the maximum yields of mutations and the integrals of the curves are the same for A and B, but occur at a less toxic dose for A than for B, then A is a more efficient mutagen than B. The kinetics of mutation and killing induction depend also on the repair processes and are sometimes very complex. In the future, such methods of analysis should be improved.

Genetic control of new substances

The majority of scientific and medical authorities who have looked into this problem, agree on the necessity of establishing a battery of tests which proceeds in progressive stages or 'tiers'. The opinions of experts (scientific or otherwise) differ about the order in which tests should be arranged, about experimental details of the protocols, and also about the persons who should be responsible for the tests.

As we have already said in several places, the number of new substances is too great to allow a systematic investigation of all possible genetic effects, and, from practical considerations, it is evident that each substance could not go through a whole battery of expensive tests.

The first fact to take into account is the real benefit of the substance under test, compared with potential risks. We have given a number of examples illustrating the concept of risks–benefits balance.

In the context of environmental mutagenesis, we have stated that it is unnecessary to continue evaluating the effects of strong agents. These are well known from much research. Either they are absolutely prescribed therapeutically, in which case there is no hesitation in accepting the risks, or they occur incidentally or accidentally in the environment, in which case all efforts should be made to detect them and minimize the risks as far as possible. For many other compounds, the problem of genetic control has not so far been easy to solve.

We proposed first to distinguish chemical classes in which different compounds have already shown high toxicity at low or very low doses. Here, mutagenicity obviously is of much less importance. It is, for example, of no consequences to learn that potassium cyanide or mercury chloride were found to be mutagenic in plants, which are resistant to high concentrations of such substances (for KCN see Kihlman *et al.*) in Kihlman, 1966, in Gen. Refs. for $HgCl_2$, see Degraeve, 1967). If such substances were to pollute the environment even at low doses, they would represent an enormous hazard for acute or chronic intoxications independently from their potential mutagenic, carcinogenic or teratogenic effects.

Second, we should consider classes of chemicals in which toxicity has never been detected, and for which the structure of functional groups does not indicate potential biological effects, with the possible exception of allergies and hypersensitivities.

Molecular homologies (Chapter 5) could provide a basis for investigations. In the case of such substances, the battery of tests could be reduced to the minimum package recommended, i.e. less expensive routine assays, just for confirmation of the data already available. For this purpose, tests with micro-organisms could be used, if not too specific, i.e. provided they do not deal with too short a part of the genome.

Between these two extremes, there are many substances for which the risks of toxicity are already well defined. For example, we can mention the case of isoniazid, which was independently investigated by various German groups of researchers (Röhrborn *et al*, 1978). This experimental model is particularly well chosen for several reasons. Former data had indicated clastogenicity in plant cells (Moutschen *et al.*, 1956), always much less than alkylating agents and acting by a different mechanism. The first observations on mouse and Chinese hamster leucocytes cultured *in vitro* revealed few clastogenic effects, and these effects were not proportional to the doses. More complete and convincing tests in mammals (dominant lethal mutations and chromosome breakage *in vivo*) generally yielded quite negative results. At that point, metabolic measurements were required, since hydrazine, one of the metabolites of isoniazid, was found to be mutagenic (Chapter 4) (review in Kimball, 1977). The circumstances in which this transformation occurs are rather exceptional, and it is not likely to happen under normal conditions of medical treatment.

Which tests remain to be done? One should first make sure that the frequency of point mutations is not increased. Also, experiments have generally been performed on males, but hazards for females should be definitely ruled out.

According to the German researchers, there is no longer any objection to using isoniazid in normal therapeutic practice, especially because of its major importance in curing severe diseases.

In recent reports, the effects of isoniazid in long-term animal bioassays were compared with short-term tests in micro-organisms (Jansen *et al.*, 1980). These studies indicate that epidemiological control of populations of patients submitted to antituberculosis treatment should be carried out.

All these observations on the genetic toxicity of isoniazid are a model of group studies. They allowed almost definitive conclusions on an important problem to be drawn after a relatively short time. There is, in fact, an historical context to this study, since isoniazid was released onto the market long before all the classicial toxicological tests had been performed, because of the urgent need for new antituberculosis drugs. Paradoxically, this may be one of the best models in genetic toxicology. Thus, in emergencies, the strategy of testing is completely reversed.

Various strategies have been proposed to assess the risks for man of different classes of substances. A procedure in three tiers was described by Bridges (1973) (Fig. 38). The first tier comprises *in vitro* tests and deals with mutations induced in bacteria, or chromosome damage induced in mammalian tissue cultures. At this stage, one or other classical *Drosophila* test could possibly be added as a valuable ancillary test. In case of negative results, these tests could be sufficient for substances with which man has only few intermittent contacts, the risk being low. In contrast, positive results would require going directly to

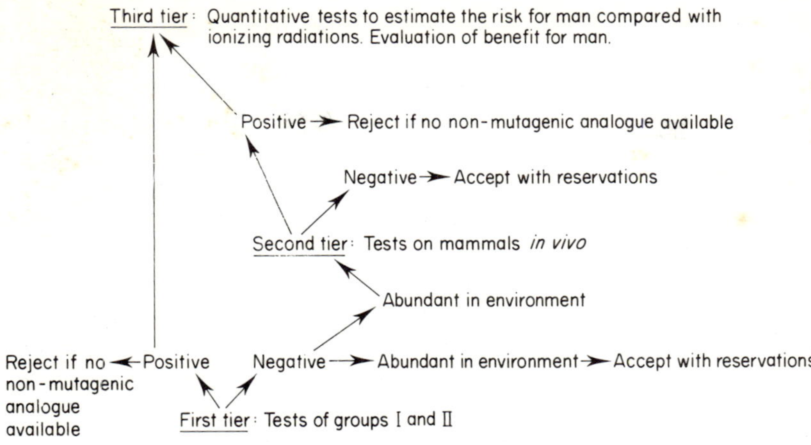

FIG. 38. Progressive tiers. (After Bridges, 1973.)

the third tier (see below).

The second tier includes *in vivo* mutagenicity tests, particularly in mammals, such as dominant lethal mutations, chromosome breakage, and possibly host-mediated assay.

On the first tier, a negative result, properly reproduced in different competent laboratories, would lead to the acceptance of the substance with some restrictions. Positive results on the second tier would lead to the rejection of the substance unless particularly important considerations warrant going on to the third tier.

This third tier would concentrate on a more quantitative toxicological evaluation of the risks for man.

Some researchers, among them Legator (quoted in Bridges, 1973), stated that *in vitro* tests of the lower tier are not sufficient by themselves and that the two upper tiers should be maintained. They upheld this opinion (Legator and Zimmering, 1975), which was also advocated by other researchers (e.g. Bochkov *et al.*, 1976; Dean, 1976; Schöneich, 1976). These researchers argued that *in vitro* test systems alone are inadequate because they are only qualitative, and that when quantitative data are required it is necessary to include *in vivo* tests at all levels, stating that it is almost a prerequisite for drawing firm conclusions. This is especially true for food additives, cosmetics, drugs, lipid-soluble pesticides and industrial chemicals (review in Rinkus and Legator, 1980).

In cases where homologous series had been previously investigated, the tests in the first tier would probably be sufficient if a good prediction could be derived from the molecular structure. This progressive procedure through the tiers sometimes runs into difficulties. First, how to choose in each tier the test most adaptable to many practical circumstances? There is as yet no general solution, and for solving urgent problems empirical decisions should be taken. An investigation of the clastogenic efficiency could in some ways be too sensitive, especially if the analysis of sister-chromatid exchanges is added. It can lead to underestimations for other types of mutations. Conversely, assays on lower organisms could overestimate the effects of point mutations, but would ignore the gross effects on chromosomes.

Now in man, like in other mammals, the chromosome structure is complex. This simple fact should be borne in mind. In the present stage of our knowledge, we think that it would be prudent to use simultaneously a sufficiently large battery of tests whenever possible, bearing in mind the cost and the number of substances needing investigation.

Schubert (1969, 1972) has already stated that no class of mutations should be neglected. According to Legator and Zimmering (1975), the selection of substances recently introduced onto the market should be based mainly on the following criteria in an attempt to avoid the long procedure described above:

(a) The use of the compound and its quantity in the environment.
(b) The relationship between structure and activity. This relationship was illustrated for various compounds with examples of homologous series (Chapter 5).
(c) The sum of results about the mutagenic activity already acquired from the literature. This latter analysis should of course be critical (see below).

This procedure will perhaps not be sufficiently efficient and complete to solve all problems in all circumstances.

An important part of mutagenetic studies, not evident from the battery of tests, involves an adequate knowledge of the metabolic pathways of the compound being investigated. Systematically, metabolic studies should be performed in parallel with the tests or sometimes even before them. These metabolic investigations are performed using multiple chemical techniques which allow detection, isolation and comparative purification of substances in the environment (Fishbein, 1972, in Gen. Refs.).

Comparative investigations on mammalian species would provide valuable information, and could be supplemented by host-mediated assays. A more precise knowledge of metabolic pathways, and of the possibilities of interactions would sometimes avoid further time-consuming and expensive analyses. In this respect, let us remember the example of the methylxanthines: caffeine, theophylline and theobromine. These substances were tested in all possible systems, and many publications were devoted to their effects. Previous knowledge of their rapid metabolism by mammalian cells under normal conditions could have served as a guideline (Chapter 4).

At the top of the battery of tests, an ultimate measure of the potential effects in man is required. Here, of course, an unbiased genetic investigation dealing with more than one generation is completely excluded. However, epidemiological studies are possible, and in Chapter 9 we emphasize the importance of prophylaxis in surveillance and monitoring of human populations.

Recently, more extreme opinions have been held about the strategy for developing the test battery. This arises from the aim to screen compounds simultaneously for both mutagenicity and carcinogenicity. According to some researchers, only short-term test systems should be developed (classified in tier 1) (review in Hollstein *et al.*, 1979). These would comprise an Ames test with and without microsomal fraction. Since this test does not allow the effects at the chromosomal level to be detected, a test with a eukaryote (e.g. yeast) should be added. Other *in vitro* tests could also be added, such as the evaluation of chromosome damage and possibly the analysis of sister-chromatid exchanges. The major argument, apart from the cost of the long-term tests, is the possibility to predict carcinogenicity if the assays are properly designed. Some researchers who advocated this procedure proposed performing additional tests specific for carcinogenicity such as mouse lymphoma or cell transformation *in vitro*.

Unfortunately, the exact relationship between *in vitro* cell transformation and cancer induction *in vivo* is far from being understood. It is certainly true that methods specifically designed for such a purpose *in vivo* are unfortunately handicapped by the very high cost, the long time needed and the expertise required of the personnel.

However, it should be borne in mind that cancer induction is a highly tissue-specific process, the complexity of which could not in any case be oversimplified. Today the consensus of opinion of scientists, and also of the medical authorities, is that critical reviews of the test systems are needed to establish new strategies for test battery development in a great variety of circumstances. Such critical reviews are part of international programmes such as the ICPEM (see Introduction) performed by groups of experienced researchers who compare the data, try to rationalize the protocols and control the reproducibility of the experiments. They may also suggest guidelines and regulations from which legal decisions could be taken.

A PROPHYLACTIC ALTERNATIVE: ANTIMUTAGENESIS

If a noxious substance is accidentally introduced into the body, the first action is to find a means of neutralizing it directly by giving an antidote. Specific antidotes could be used not only in the case of acute accidents but also after long-term occupational exposure to potential mutagens. Such substances designed to counteract the action of mutagens could be named *antimutagens*.

The concept of antimutagenicity was first proposed by Westergaard (1957). He mentioned that catalase inhibitors could produce mutations. These inhibitors act in an indirect manner by accumulating hydrogen peroxide, a well-known mutagen (Chapters 4 and 6).

Conversely, increased catalase activity would be expected to decrease the risk of damage from hydrogen peroxide since a faster detoxification would not allow the threshold of activity to be reached.

Generally, with adaptive enzymes working in the same way, it is of importance one way or another not to interfere with normal functions. Whatever the mechanism(s) of action, it is known that various substances can either strongly decrease or even completely prevent mutagenic action, as is the case for some purine nucleosides such as adenosine, guanosine and inosine ribonucleosides in *E. coli*. This antimutagenic property is somewhat specific. For instance, these substances act against trimethylxanthines and some purine derivatives such as azaguanine. In contrast, the frequency of mutations due to UV light, benzimidazole and tetramethyluric acid is not modified (Figs. 39 and 40).

The mechanisms responsible for this antimutagenicity are not yet well elucidated. Paradoxically, quinacrine, a mutagenic and clastogenic substance in several organisms (Chapter 5), decreases the frequency of spontaneous, or induced mutations in two strains in which a high frequency of mutations due to the mutators (*mut T* and *ast-I*) is observed (Zamenhof, 1969). This observation should be of some practical interest in determining in what circumstances quinacrine and other acridine derivatives show antimutagenicity.

Another substance, spermine, a polyamine, is worth mentioning here. It strongly decreases the frequency of spontaneous or induced mutations in *mut T* or *ast-I* of *E. coli* and in *Staphylococcus aureus*. Moreover, it is active towards mutations induced by caffeine and UV light in *E. coli* UC 879 (Johnson and Bach, 1965).

At active antimutagen doses these amines are generally devoid of genotoxic effects, though chromosome damage was reported in plants with another amine: putrescine (Oehlkers, 1953). This research should be repeated with other test systems to check if such antimutagenic properties can be extended to higher organisms, and also which mutagenic effects can be modified. One should also verify that the antimutagenic activity of a substance does not result in a shift of the mutation spectrum, suppressing certain types of mutations, but favouring the expression of other types potentially more deleterious. This is

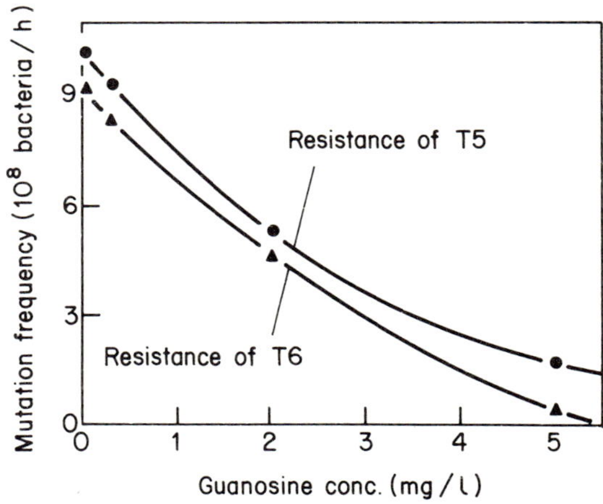

FIG. 39. Effects of increased concentrations of guanosine on the mutation frequency of *E. coli* for resistance of strains T5 and T6 induced by theophylline (150 mg/l). (After Novick, 1957.)

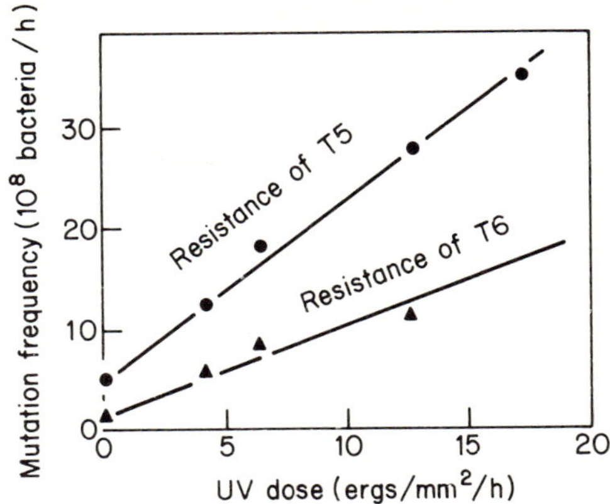

FIG. 40. Effects of increased intensity of UV light on the mutation frequency of *E. coli* for resistance of strains T5 and T6 growing on media containing tryptophan as growth factor. (After Novick, 1957.)

precisely what has been observed with cysteamine and glutathione. These efficient radioprotective substances decrease the chromosome damage induced by ionizing radiations (Mikaelsen, 1952; Moutschen, 1960). But this radioprotective effect allows a larger proportion of the irradiated cell population to survive with the subsequent occurrence of point mutations which have a higher chance of being inherited than gross chromosome damage (Kaplan and Lyon, 1953a, b; Möes, 1957).

It is tempting to imagine the possibility of synthesizing new molecules potentially active towards a large number of mutagenic agents.

A quite different antimutagenic effect than the one described above has been reported by Vogel (1973). This is the inhibition of the effects of Trenimon, a strong alkylating agent of the imine group, and to a lesser extent of 1-phenyl-3,3-dimethyltriazine by sodium fluoride in *Drosophila*. This antimutagenic property of sodium fluoride should not be generalized. With the same compound and in the same test system, Mukherjee and Sobels (1968) obtained an increase in the mutagenic effects of an acute X-ray dose of 2000 R.

The mechanism of inhibition of alkylating agents should be carefully investigated. Otherwise, the antidote could be more noxious than the poison itself, as is sometimes the case in classical toxicology.

A class of antimutagenic substances recently discovered acts by a quite indirect mechanism. The urine of two non-human primates who were treated with an antischistosomal drug, amoscanate (Chapter 4), was found to be mutagenic in an Ames test (Batzinger *et al.*, 1979). Since this drug did not show any direct mutagenic effects in the same test, it was inferred that metabolic activation had occurred somewhere. The role of intestinal micro-organisms was strongly suspected since faecal extracts made the *in vitro* test positive. Moreover, when erythromycin was given simultaneously, the mutagenic activation was prevented. Further research demonstrated that various species of *Streptococcus* are actually responsible for the transformation, and that only a very small amount of the intestinal flora is required for activation (Molineaux *et al.*, 1980).

Other antibiotics act as antimutagenic substances in the same way as erythromycin. The mechanism of action of these antibiotics is obviously by killing the activating bacteria. Since there are no direct interactions between antibiotics and amoscanate, there is no decrease of the antischistosomal activity. If these antibiotics can be used in the future at concentrations which do not generate new hazards, this finding and others along the same line of research will result in important applications in therapeutics.

Recently the concept of antimutagenicity has been somewhat enlarged. One can delineate two levels of action capable of practical application. Kada (1982) proposed to distinguish first those agents that interact directly with environmental mutagens *in vitro*. He called these agents *desmutagens* (name proposed by Drake, quoted in Kada, 1982). The second type comprises agents which interfere with cellular metabolic processes *in vivo* by various mechanisms not always elucidated.

To the first class of agents belong some compounds that are able to antagonize the mutagenic effects of tryptophan pyrolysates in cooked food (Kada *et al.*, 1978; Morita *et al.*, 1978; Sugimura, 1979; Stich *et al.*, 1982). Some researchers realized the complexity of these mutagenic processes (Stich *et al.*, 1982). To give a few examples: such food components as chlorophyll, naturally occurring antioxidants and even some trace of metals can in specific environmental conditions modify the genotoxicity of foods, acting as antimutagens. However, in other circumstances, the same factors can enhance the mutagenic effects of food components, thereby becoming the 'murderer accomplices'.

The need for controlling the activity of environmental mutagens by neutralizing their potentialities has been pointed out several times. Alekperov (1982) emphasized the importance of substances intended to decontaminate the environment being ubiquitous. Substances such as β-carotene, vitamins E and C, occurring universally, can be used in practical circumstances. Now, some of these substances are themselves mutagenic at doses at which they would be expected to show antimutagenic properties.

It seems to be a vicious circle which must be broken in the future. There are also curious examples of natural antimutagenic substances. Among these substances, the so-called 'cabbage factor' decreases mutagenic action at the Trp-P2 of *E. coli* by inactivating mutagens either directly or indirectly by inhibiting the activation of promutagens into mutagens in the microsomal fractions. On the other hand, true mutagenic substances are also known to occur in cabbages. Substances with antimutagenic potential have been described in camellia extracts (Kada, 1982). Since camellia is used for preparing green and black teas, the risks of the purine derivatives should be compared with the benefit of antimutagenic substances. It seems that nature itself wanted to put the poison and the antidote in the same place. (See also mutagenicity of naturally occurring substances in Chapter 4.)

To the second class of antimutagens, those acting at the cellular level, belong interesting substances able to reduce the frequency of induced mutations. The finding that mammalian tissue extracts possess antimutagenic properties is certainly relevant. It is known that extracts of normal placenta decrease the frequency of UV-induced mutations (reversions) in *E. coli* (Kada, 1982). Komura *et al.* (1981) considered that cobalt ions might be the major factor responsible for the antimutagenic effects. This confirmed the results found in previous research with cobalt chloride. More and more possibilities of antimutagenicity emerge as an alternative prophylactic solution to the systematic screening of all substances entering the environment in order to prevent their effects. But how to know what to prevent?

ULTIMATE RESORTS

For some decades, it held that genetic damage is irreversible, and that the accumulation of lesions leads inevitably to genetic death (Chapter 6). Today, we are aware that efficient repair processes are unceasingly at work at all levels. However, when these processes are overloaded or when they are mistaken, genetic lesions are established. Consequently, in the future, advantage should be taken of the existence of such processes in the prevention of inherited diseases, which should be better understood in order to avoid their inhibition and possibly to stimulate them. If properly handled future prophylaxis should be able to reduce the 'genetic load' of human populations.

Now, once it is identified, is there anything more that can be attempted to eradicate a genetic lesion?

The first prescribed eugenic action would be to prevent the spreading of the 'deleterious gene' in populations. This eugenic attitude, however, increasingly accepted in our modern society, is running into a great deal of practical, legal and ethical difficulties.

'Genetic therapeutics' remains an ultimate possibility. We can distinguish two possibilities. One is *gene therapy*, which means the replacement of a defective gene, such as the gene which produces a hormone in somatic cells. The other is *gene surgery*, which implies intervention in the human germ cells affecting not only the individual but also its progeny. These two possibilities are more than an auxiliary therapy in which a molecule is continuously given to a patient unable to synthesize it, like, for instance, insulin in diabetes mellitus.

As stated above, one could imagine replacing selectively and definitively the wrong 'piece of chromosome', as one might do in a car engine. The proposed substances might be highly specific mutagenic substances inducing back-mutation of the 'sick gene', or specific DNA recombinants. 'Genetic surgery', as Muller named it, is probably far from being accepted (Muller cited in Sonneborn, 1965, in Gen. Refs.). He has listed the many genetic objections resulting from the application of such a procedure. If we imagine that we could without hazard induce a specific genetic change, it remains to discover where to operate after knowing the relation between the inherited defect and its genetic cause.

It should be remembered that a large majority of genetic diseases in man, inherited syndromes, are quite complex. On the one hand, various disorders with almost the same phenotype arise from lesions located in different parts of chromosomes or even in different chromosomes. On the other hand, in the same disorder, several regions of chromosomes may be simultaneously involved. Only in rare cases of very simple genetic diseases can the exact chromosomal region responsible be unmistakenly identified, and thereafter the difficulty of the 'surgical' operation remains enormous.

The possibility of identifying genes by genetic manipulations involving cloning genes inside bacteria, and by molecular hybridization of nucleic acids gives new insights. Although from the present viewpoint, this method is still in quite an early stage, it is fast progressing.

According to Muller, the wise solution lies in the present and not in a remote and problematic future. It matters to prevent the degeneration of human populations by avoiding the spread of genetic diseases. Muller even goes one step further when he states that we should 'transcend our stone age genetic constitutions by adapting to the requirement of our atomic age'.

However, it is a matter of course that the 'germinal choice' recommended by Muller raises multiple ethical problems. They might be solved at least partly by improving our knowledge of human inheritance.

It is imperative to be fully conscious of the work to do, and to apply ourselves urgently and eagerly to the task.

Glossary

Alkylating agent: substance reacting with DNA by a process of alkylation (introduction of alkyl groups) hence producing mutations.

Allele (or allelomorph): one of a pair of characters alternative to each other, being governed by loci located at homologous sites on homologous chromosomes.

Aneuploid: an organism or cells not possessing the exact chromosome number (= partially polyploid).

Antimitotic (substance): a substance which inhibits mitosis in a reversible or non-reversible way.

Autosome: chromosome which is not a sex (X or Y) chromosome.

Auxotroph: mutant (generally in lower organisms) growing only on supplemented medium, which is required for achieving its biological cycle.

Auxotrophy: quality of an auxotrophic mutant.

Chimaera: organism composed of tissues of two or more genetically distinct types.

Chloroplast: intracellular plant organelle containing several pigments (including chlorophyll). This organelle is the site of photosynthesis.

Clastogenicity: chromosome breakage. Many compounds are clastogenic, i.e. induce chromosome damage.

Colchicomitosis: abnormal mitosis produced by colchicine (alkaloid extracted from the autumn crocus, *Colchicum autumnale*) or by substances having similar cytological effects. Spindle fibres are suppressed so chromosomes cannot move towards the poles and polyploid cells (see under *polyploid*) can result.

Conidia: spores ensuring asexual propagation of fungi.

Constriction (chromosomic): an uncoiled chromosomic segment of fixed position. Primary constrictions are centromeres. Secondary constrictions separate satellites from the rest of the chromosomes. Some organize the nucleolus (nucleolar constrictions). Tertiary constrictions are located at sites different from primary and secondary constrictions.

Conversion (genic): error produced in gene copy at the time of replication, generally meiosis.

Convertogenic substance: one that induces conversion.

Corpora lutea: yellow glandular bodies formed from Graafian follicles after extrusion of ova from mammalian ovaries. In mutagenicity tests such as dominant lethal mutation assays, corpora lutea must be distinguished from those induced during pregnancy.

Crossing-over: reciprocal exchange of homologous chromatids from homologous chromosomes. This exchange, naturally occurring at meiosis, can also be observed, but more rarely, in any cell (somatic crossing-over).

Deciduoma: word used in the dominant lethal mutation assay, as synonymous with embryo deaths.

Deficiency: loss of a terminal segment of chromosome.

Deletion: loss of an internal segment of chromosome.

Dicentric: abnormal chromosome with two centromeres.

Diploid: the normal somatic number of chromosomes ($2n$), one set from each parent.

Dominant character: that possessed by one parent and appearing at the first generation (F_1) to the exclusion of the allelic character from the other parent. Dominance can be complete, incomplete or absent.

Duplication: occurrence of one chromosomic segment twice in the same chromosome complement.

Embryo sac: female gametophyte of higher plants arising from the macrospore (see under *macrospore*).

Endopolyploidy: repeated division of the chromosomes without nuclear and cellular divisions.

Endosperm: triploid nutritive tissue of a seed arising from double fertilization, from the fusion of the second nucleus of the pollen cell and two of the eight nuclei of the embryo sac (see also *embryo sac*).

Endospore: uni- or multicellular capsulated spore.

Fluorochrome (or fluor): fluorescent dye such as acridine orange, fluorescein isothiocyanate.

Gamete: cell of meiotic origin generally produced in sexual organs and capable of fertilization.

Genome: complete chromosome set of a gamete (= chromosome complement).

Genome mutation: modification of the normal genome number, as in the case of polyploidy (see *polyploidy*).

Genotype: entire genetic constitution of the organism, expressed or latent.

Gonad: organ in which spermatozoa or ova are formed (testes and ovaries).

Haploid: complete set of chromosomes as found in gametes.

Hemizygous: a gene with no allele, being in an unpaired state as in a haploid organism, or unpaired sex chromosome as in a diploid organism (see X chromosome).

Heteroploidy: a polyploidy in which the chromosome number is not an exact multiple of the basic haploid number.

Heterozygous: organism arising fromt he gametic fusion of dissimilar genetic constitutions.

Homozygous: organism with one or more gene(s) present in the double condition.

Karyotype: chromosome complement characteristic of a group or taxonomic unit.

Lethal gene: one which in the homozygous state leads inevitably to the death of the carrier. When homozygotes are capable of surviving for a rather long period, the gene is called sublethal, semilethal or subviable.

Linkage: association of genes of the same chromosome.

Locus: the fixed position of the gene in the chromosome.

Macrospore (or megaspore): the cell which, in higher plants, gives rise to the embryo sac.

Meiosis: succession of two cell divisions occurring in sexual organs, in which the number of chromosomes is reduced from the diploid number ($2n$) to the haploid (n).

Microsomal: subcellular fraction isolated by differential centrifugation containing two components: (1) a membranous or endoplasmic reticulum; (2) a ribosomal fraction active in protein synthesis.

Mitosis: somatic cell division resulting in two daughter cells with normally equivalent genomes, it comprises prophase, metaphase, anaphase, and telophase.

Mutation: any sudden change of the genotype.

Mutation rate: frequency at which mutations occur in an organism.

Mycelium: the entirety of ramified threads forming the vegetative apparatus of a fungus.

Non-disjunction: (chromosome): failure of paired chromosomes to separate at meiosis so that both enter the same daughter nucleus which will have one more chromosome, the other daughter nucleus lacking one chromosome.

Oogensis: formation of ova from stem cells. This comprises successive stages: oogonia, oocytes I and II (involving meiosis), oocids and ova. This process occurs in ovary.

Ovum: female gamete.

Phenotype: group of individuals with the same appearance (as opposed to genotype; see this word).

Pleiotropism (pleiotropy): a gene governing more than one character.

Polygene: this word has two concepts: (1) a set of linked genes (see *linkage*) determining quantitative characters; (2) a set of minor genes not necessarily linked, also determining quantitative characters such as weight, height.

Polyploid: organism or parts of an organism whose somatic nuclei contain more than two sets of chromosomes, i.e. with a higher chromosome number than the diploid.

Promutagen: substance that is not directly mutagenic by itself, but which can be activated into a real mutagen (ultimate mutagen) either in the environment or in the body.

Radiomimetic: a substance that has cytotoxic or mutagenic effects comparable in some ways to the effects of ionizing radiations.

Recombination: rearrangement of linked genes due to crossing-over (*see* crossing-over).

Recombinogenic: substance that modifies the crossing-over processes and, therefore, the frequency of recombinations.

Sex-linked (characters): association between these characters and sex chromosomes (see X and Y).

Somatic mutation: a mutation in somatic (body) cells which may or may not result in a chimaera (*see* Chimaera).

Spermatogenesis: formation of spermatozoa from stem cells. This comprises successive stages: spermatogonia, spermatocytes I and II (involving meiosis), spermatids and spermatozoa. This process occurs in the testis.

Syndrome: a set of symptoms characteristic of a disease even if the origin is unknown.

Transforming factor: DNA extracted from a bacterial strain (donor) capable of transforming another strain (receptor), for example in *Pneumococcus*, in which transforming factor can transform smooth strain into rough.

Trisomy: the state in which organisms or cells have one or more chomosomes present three times instead of twice.

X (chromosome): sex pairing with its homologous chromosome in the homozygous sex (female in mammals) or with a not completely homologous chromosome (Y chromosome) in the heterozygous sex (male in mammals).

Y (*see* X chromosome)

Zygote: cell resulting from fusion of gametes.

References

Textbooks, Monographs, Handbooks, Proceedings of Symposia, Series and Reviews of more general interest

Auerbach, C. (1976) *Mutation Research. Problems, results and perspectives*. Chapman and Hall (London).

Bacq, Z.M., and Alexander, P. (1955) *Principes de Radiobiologie*. Sciences et Lettres (Liège) and Masson (Paris).

Bauer, K.H. (1928) *Mutationstheorie der Geschwulst-Entstehung. Übergang von Körperzellen in Geschwulstzellen durch Gen-Änderung*. Springer-Verlag (Berlin).

Boveri, T. (1929) *The Origin of Malignant Tumors*. Williams and Wilkins (Baltimore).

Burdette, W. (1962) *Methodology in Human Genetics*. Holden-Day (San Francisco).

Burdette, W. (1963a) *Methodology in Basic Genetics*. Holden-Day (San Francisco).

Burdette, W. (1963b) *Methodology in Mammalian Genetics*. Holden-Day (San Francisco).

Butterworth, B.E., and Goldberg, L. (1979) *Strategies for Short-term Testing Mutagens/Carcinogens*. CRC Press (West Palm Beach, Florida).

de Serres, F.J. (ed.) (1983) *Chemical Mutagens. Principles and Methods for their Detection*, Vol. 8. Plenum Press (New York and London).

de Serres, F.J., and Hollaender, A. (eds.) (1980) *Chemical Mutagens. Principles and Methods for their Detection*, Vol. 6. Plenum Press (New York and London).

de Serres, F.J., and Hollaender, A. (eds.) (1982) *Chemical Mutagens. Principles and Methods for their Detection*, Vol. 7. Plenum Press (New York and London).

de Serres, F.J., Fouts, J.R., Bend, J.R., and Philpot, R.M. (1976) *In Vitro Metabolic Activation in Mutagenesis Testing*. North-Holland (Amsterdam, New York, Oxford).

Dobzhansky, Th. (1957) *Genetics and the Origin of Species* (3rd revised edition). Columbia University Press (New York).

Ehrenberg, L., and Gustafsson, Å. (1970) *Chemical Mutagens: Their Uses and Hazards in Medicine and Technology*, National Board of Health Report, Sweden, in Swedish and English. Carl Bloms Boktryckeri (Lund).

Epstein, S.S., and Legator, M.S. (1971) *The Mutagenicity of Pesticides. Concepts and Evaluation*. MIT Press (Cambridge, MA.

Evans, H.J. (1962) Chromosome aberrations induced by ionizing radiations. *Int. Rev. Cytol.*, **13**, 221–321.

First International Conference on Environmental Mutagens, *(Asilomar, Pacific Grove, CA* (1973).

Fishbein, L. (1972) *Chromatography of Environmental Hazards,* Vol. 1. Elsevier (Amsterdam)

Fishbein, L., Flamm, W.G. and Falk, H.L. (1970) *Chemical Mutagens: Environmental Effects on Biological Systems — Environmental Sciences*. An interdisciplinary monograph series. Academic Press (New York and London).

Frankel, O.H., and Bennett, E. (1970) *Genetic Resources in Plants. Their Exploration and Conservation*. Blackwell Scientific Publications (Oxford).

Gustafsson, Å. (1947) Mutation in agricultural plants. *Hereditas*, **33**, 1–100.

Hagberg, A., and Åkerberg, E. (1962) *Mutations and Polyploidy in Plant Breeding*. Svenska Bokförlaget Bonniers (Stockholm).

Hollaender, A. (1954) *Radiation Biology*, Vol. I, Parts I and II, McGraw-Hill (New York, Toronto and London).

Hollaender, A. (ed.) (1955) *Radiation Biology*. Vol. II, McGraw-Hill (New York, Toronto and London).
Hollaender, A. (ed.) (1971a) *Chemical Mutagens. Principles and Methods for their Detection*, Vol. 1. Plenum Press (New York and London).
Hollaender, A. (ed.) (1971b) *Chemical Mutagens. Principles and Methods for their Detection*, Vol. 2. Plenum Press (New York and London).
Hollaender, A. (ed.) (1973) *Chemical Mutagens. Principles and Methods for their Detection*, Vol. 3. Plenum Press (New York and London).
Hollaender, A. (ed.) (1976) *Chemical Mutagens. Principles and Methods for their Detection*, Vol. 4. Plenum Press (New York and London).
Hollaender, A., and de Serres, F.J. (1978) *Chemical Mutagens. Principles and Methods for their Detection*, Vol. 5. Plenum Press (New York and London).
ICPEMC International Commission for Protection against Environmental Mutagens and Carcinogens. See publications and working papers in *Mutat. Res.,* **54**, 3 (1978) and following.
Kihlman, B. (1966) *Actions of Chemicals on Dividing Cells*. Prentice-Hall (Englewood Cliffs, NJ).
Kilbey, B.J., Legator, M., Nichols, W., and Ramel, C. (1977) *Handbook of Mutagenicity Test Procedures*. Elsevier (Amsterdam).
Kirsch-Volders, M. (ed.) (1984) *Mutagenicity, Carcinogenicity and Teratogenicity of Industrial Pollutants*. Plenum Press (New York and London.
Lewis, K.R., and John, B. (1963) *Chromosome Marker*. Churchill (London).
Malling, H.V., and de Serres, F.J. (1971) *A Laboratory Manual for the Use of Neurospora in the Host-mediated Assay in Tests for Mutagenicity*. Workshop of Mutagenicity, Brown University (Providence, Rhode Island).
Mather, K. (1949) *Biometrical Genetics*. Dover Publications (New York).
Meier, H. (1963) *Experimental Pharmacogenetics. Physiopathology of Heredity and Pharmacologic Responses*. Academic Press (New York and London).
Moorhead, P.S. (1970) *Genetic Concept and Neoplasia*. Williams and Wilkins (Baltimore).
Moutschen, J. (1965) Les effets cytogénétiques des composés alkane sulfonates d'alkyl. *Mém. Soc. R. Sci. Liège*, **11**, 296.
Mutation and Plant Breeding (Symposium on), *Nat. Acad. Sci., Nat. Res. Counc.* (Washington), Publ. 891: 523 pp (1961).
Nilan, R.A. (1964) *The Cytology and Genetics of Barley*, 1951–1962. Monogr. Suppl. No 3, Res. Stud., Washington State Univ. Press (Pullman), vol. 32, No 1: 278 pp. (1964).
Peters, R.A. (1952) Lethal syntheses. *Proc. R. Soc. Ser. B.*, **139**, 143–170.
Ramade, F. (1974) *Eléments d'Écologie Appliquée*. Ediscience — McGraw-Hill (Paris).
Ramel, C (1973) Evaluation of genetic risks of environmental chemicals. *Ambio Special Report*, **3**, 1–27.
Rieger, R., and Michaelis, A. (1967) Die Chromosomenmutationen. In *Genetik: Grundlagen, Ergebnisse und Probleme in Einzeldarstellungen*, Beitrag 6. Gustav Fischer Verlag (Iena).
Ross, W.C.J. (1962) *Biological Alkylating Agents. Fundamental Chemistry and the Design of Compounds for Selective Toxicity*. Butterworths (London).
Scott, D., Bridges, B.A., and Sobels, F.H. (1977) *Progress in Genetic Toxicology*. Elsevier/North-Holland (Amsterdam).
Sonneborn, T.M. (1965) *The Control of Human Heredity and Evolution*. Macmillan (New York).
Stebbins, G.L. (1957) *Variation and Evolution in Plants*, 3rd edition, Columbia University Press (New York).
Sugimura, T., Kondo, S., and Takebe, H. (eds.) (1982) Environmental mutagens and carcinogens. *Proceedings 3rd International Conference on Environmental Mutagens,*

Tokyo, Mishima and Kyoto, September 21–27, 1981. University of Tokyo Press (Tokyo) and Alan R. Liss (New York).

Sutton, H.E., and Harris, M.I. (1972) *Mutagenic Effects of Environmental Contaminants*. Academic Press (New York).

Swanson, C.P. (1957) *Cytology and Cytogenetics: some aberrations*. Prentice-Hall (Englewood Cliffs, NJ).

UNSCEAR (1972) *A report of the United Nations scientific committee on the effects of atomic radiation*. General assembly, with annexes vol. II (A 8725) 27th Session, Suppl. No 25, United Nations (New York).

Vavilov, N.I. (1949/50) The origin, variation, immunity and breeding of cultivated plants (selected papers translated from Russian by K. Starr Chester). *Chron. Bot.* **13**, 1–264.

Vogel, F., and Röhrborn, G. (1970) *Chemical Mutagenesis in Mammals and Man*. Springer-Verlag (Berlin, Heidelberg and New York).

Wright, S. (1968) *Evolution and the Genetics of Populations*, Vol. 1. University of Chicago Press (Chicago).

Wright, J.W., and Pal, R. (1967) *Genetics of Insect Vectors of Disease*. Elsevier (Amsterdam).

References to Introduction

Loprieno, N. (1983) Control of commercial chemicals, the sixth amendment to the directive on dangerous chemical substances (79/831/EEC) adopted by the Council of the European Communities. In Chemical Mutagens (see de Serres in Gen. Refs.) Vol. 8, pp. 343–366.

Public Law 94–469–Oct., 1976–94th Congress. Appendix in *Chemical Mutagens* (see Hollaender and de Serres in Gen. Refs.) Vol. 5, pp. 287–335 (1978).

Sanders, H.J. (1969) Chemical mutagens. The road to genetic disaster? *Chem. Eng. News*, **47**, 50–65, 71.

Sobels, F.H. (1977) The founding of the International Commission for Protection against Environmental Mutagens and Carcinogens (ICPEMC). In *Progress in Genetic Toxicology* (see Scott *et al.* in Gen. Refs.), pp. 117–121.

Sobels, F.H., and Delehanty, J. (1982) The first five years of ICPEMC, The International Commission for Protection against Environmental Mutagens and Carcinogens. In *Environmental Mutagens and Carcinogens* (see Sugimura *et al.* in Gen. Refs.) pp. 81–90.

References to Chapter 1

Ames, B.N., Durston, W.E., Yamasaki, E., and Lee, F.D. (1973) Carcinogens are mutagens: a simple test system combining liver homogenates for activation and bacteria for detection. *Proc. Natl. Acad. Sci. USA*, **70**, 2281–2285.

Ames, B.N., McCann, J., and Yamasaki, E. (1975) Methods for detecting carcinogens and mutagens with the *Salmonella*/mammalian microsome mutagenicity test. *Mutat. Res.*, **31**, 347–364.

Ansari, A.A., and Malling, H.V. (1982) The use of immunological techniques to detect cells of rare genotype. In *Chemical Mutagens* (see de Serres and Hollaender in Gen. Refs.), Vol. 7, pp. 37–87.

Bailey, P.W., (1979) An assay for histocompatibility gene mutations in mice. *Genetics*, **92**, S59–S62 (Suppl.).

Bridges, B.A. (1980) The fluctuation test. *Arch. Toxicol.*, **46**, 41–44.

Brink, R.A., and MacGillivray, J.H. (1924) Segregation for the *waxy* character in maize pollen and differential development of the male gametophyte. *Am. J. Bot.*, **11**, 465–469.

Brookes, P., and Lawley, P.D. (1964) Evidence for binding of polynuclear aromatic hydrocarbons and their binding to DNA. *Nature*, **202**, 781–784.

Chu, E.H.Y. (1970) Point mutations in mammalian cell cultures as measures for mutagenicity testing. In *Chemical Mutagenesis in Mammals and Man* (see Vogel and Röhrborn in Gen. Refs.); pp. 241–250.

Chu, E.H.Y. (1971) Induction and analysis of gene mutations in mammalian cells in culture. In *Chemical Mutagens* (see Hollaender in Gen. Refs.), Vol. 2, 411–444.

Chu, E.H.Y., and Malling, H.V. (1968a) Chemical mutagenesis in Chinese hamster cells *in vivo*. *Proc. XII Int. Congr. Genet., (Tokyo),* **1**, 102 (Abstract).

Chu, E.H.Y., and Malling, H.V. (1968b) Mammalian cell genetics. II. Chemical induction of specific locus mutations in Chinese hamster cells *in vitro*. *Proc. Natl. Acad. Sci. USA*, **61**, 1302–1312.

Chu, E.H.Y., and Malling, H.V. (1971) Induction of mutations in mammalian cells implanted in heterologous hosts. *2nd Annu. Meet. Environ. Mutagen Soc. (Zinkovy)*, pp. 11–12 (abstract).

Cleaver, J.E. (1968) Defective repair replication of DNA in Xeroderma pigmentosum. *Nature*, **218**, 652–656.

Cleaver, J.E. (1969) Xeroderma pigmentosum: A human disease in which an initial stage of DNA repair is defective. *Proc. Natl. Acad. Sci. USA* **63**, 428–435.

Cole, J., Arlett, C.F., and Green, M.H.L. (1976) The fluctuation test as a more sensitive system for determining induced mutation in L5178Y mouse lymphoma cells. *Mutat. Res.*, **41**, 377–386.

Demerec, M. (1924) A case of pollen dimorphism in maize. *Am. J. Bot.*, **11**, 461–464.

Ehrenberg, L., and Eriksson, G. (1966) The dose dependence of mutation rates in the rad range, in the light of experiments with higher plants. *Acta Radiol. (Suppl.)*, **254,** 73–81.

Ehrenberg, L., and Osterman-Golkar, S. (1980) Alkylation of macromolecules for detecting mutagenic agents. *Teratogenesis, Carcinogenesis, Mutagenesis,* **1**, 105–127.

Eriksson, G. (1962) Radiation-induced reversions of a *waxy* allele in barley. *Radiat. Bot.*, **2**, 35–39.

Eriksson, G. (1969) The *waxy* character. *Hereditas*, **63**, 180–204.

Fahrig, R. (1971) Metabolic activation of aryldialkyltriazenes in the mouse: induction of mitotic gene conversion in *Saccharomyces cerevisiae* in the host-mediated assay. *Mutat. Res.*, **13**, 436–439.

Gabridge, M.G., and Legator, M.S. (1969) A host-mediated microbial assay for the detection of mutagenic compounds. *Proc. Soc. Exp. Biol. Med.*, **130**, 831–834.

Gabridge, M.G., De Nunzio, A., and Legator, M.S. (1969) Microbial mutagenicity of streptozotocin in animal mediated assays. *Nature*, **221**, 68.

Gatehouse, D.G., and Delow, G.F. (1979) The development of a 'Microtitre K' fluctuation test for the detection of indirect mutagens and its use in the evaluation of mixed enzyme induction of the liver. *Mutat. Res.*, **60**, 239–252.

Green, M.H.L., Bridges, B.A., Rogers, A.M., Horspool, G., Muriel W.J., Bridges, J.W., and Fry, J.R. (1977) Mutagen screening by a simplified fluctuation test: use of microsomal preparations and whole liver cells for metabolic activation. *Mutat. Res.*, **48,** 287–294.

Hofnung, M., and Weil, N. (1980) Inductest and spermatest in genetic toxicology testing. *Arch. Toxicol.*, **46,** 159–169.

Hubbard, S.A., Green, M.H.L., Bridges, B.A., Wain, A.J., and Bridges, J.W. (1980) The fluctuation test with S9 and hepatocyte activation. In *Short Term Tests for Carcinogenicity.*, Report of the International Collaborative Programme eds. F.H. de Serres and J. Ashby. Elsevier/North-Holland (Amsterdam).

Ichikawa, S., and Sparrow, A.H. (1968) The use of induced somatic mutations to study cell division rates in irradiated stamen hairs of *Tradescantia virginiana* L., *Jap.J. Genet.*, **43,** 57–63.

Ichikawa, S., Sparrow, A.H., and Thompson, K.H. (1969) Morphologically abnormal cells, somatic mutations and loss of reproductive integrity in irradiated *Tradescantia* stamen hairs. *Radiat. Bot.*, **9,** 195–211.

Kao, F.T., and Puck, T.T. (1968a) *Isolation of nutritionally deficient mutants of Chinese hamster cells.* Proc. XII Int. Congr. Genet. (Tokyo) **1,** 157 (Abstract).

Kao, F.T., and Puck, T.T. (1968b) Genetics of somatic mammalian cells. VII. Induction and isolation of nutritional mutants in Chinese hamster cells. *Proc. Natl. Acad. Sci USA.*, **60,** 1275–1281.

Klein J. (1978) *H*-2 mutations: Their genetics and effect on immune functions. *Adv. Immunol.*, **26**, 55–146.

Kohn, K.W., and Grimek-Ewig, R.A. (1973) Alkaline elution analysis, a new approach to the study of DNA single-strand interruptions in cells. *Cancer Res.*, **33**, 1849–1853.

Kohn, H.I., and Melvold, R.W. (1974) Spontaneous histocompatibility mutations detected by dermal grafts: significant changes in rate over a 10-year period in the mouse H-system. *Mutat. Res.*, **24,** 163–169.

Krooth, R.S., Darlington, G.A., and Velazquez, A.A. (1968) The genetics of cultured mammalian cells. *Annu. Rev. Genet.*, **2,** 141–164.

Lederberg, J., and Lederberg, E.M. (1952) Replica plating and indirect selection of bacterial mutants. *J. Bacteriol.*, **63,** 399–406.

Lee, I.P., and Zbinden, G. (1979) Differential DNA damage induced by chemical mutagens in cells growing in a modified Selye's granuloma pouch. *Exp. Cell Biol.*, **47,** 92–106.

Legator, M.S. (1970) The host-mediated assay, a practical procedure for evaluating potential mutagenic agents. In *Chemical Mutagenesis in Mammals and Man* (see Vogel and Röhrborn in Gen. Refs.) pp. 260–270.

Longley, A.F. (1924) Chromosomes in maize and relatives. *J. Agric. Res.*, **28,** 673–681.

Luria, S.E., and Delbrück, M. (1943) Mutations of bacteria from virus sensitivity to virus resistance. *Genetics,* **28,** 491–511.

Lutz, W.K. (1979) *In vivo* covalent binding of organic chemicals to DNA as a quantitative indicator in the process of chemical carcinogenesis. *Mutat. Res.*, **65,** 289–356.

Malling, H.V., and Cosgrove, G.E. (1970) The internal level of mutagens in mammals. In *Chemical Mutagenesis in Mammals and Man* (see Vogel and Röhrborn in Gen. Refs.), pp. 271–278.

Marmur, J. (1961) A procedure for the isolation of deoxyribonucleic acid from micro-organisms. *J. Mol. Biol.*, **3,** 208–218.

McCann, J., Choi, E., Yamasaki, E., and Ames, B.N. (1975) Detection of carcinogens as mutagens in the *Salmonella* microsome test: assay of 300 chemicals. *Proc. Natl. Acad. Sci USA,* **72**, 5135–5139.

Melchers, F., Potter, M., and Warner, N.L. (eds.) (1978) *Curr. Top. Microbiol. Immuno.* **81.**

Mohn, G.R. (1981) Bacterial systems for carcinogenicity testing. *Mutat. Res.*, **87,** 191–210.

Montesano, R., and Magee, P.N. (1970) Metabolism of dimethylnitrosamine by human liver slices *in vitro. Nature,* **228,** 173.

Moustachi, E. (1980) Mutagenicity testing with eukaryotic micro-organisms. *Arch. Toxicol.*, **46,** 99–110.

Nelson, O.E. (1957) The feasibility of investigating 'genetic fine structure' in higher plants. *Am. Nat.*, **91,** 331–332.

Nelson, O.E. (1968) The *waxy* locus in maize. II. The location of the controlling elements alleles. *Genetics,* **60,** 507–524.

Parry, J.M. (1977) The use of yeast cultures for the detection of environmental mutagens using a fluctuation test. *Mutat. Res.*, **46**, 165–176.

Rosichan, J.L., Arenay, P., Blake, N., Hodjdon, A., Kleinhofs, A., and Nilan, R.A. (1981) An improved method for the detection of mutants at the *waxy* locus in *Hordeum vulgare. Environ. Mutagenesis,* **8,** 91–93.

Sega, G.A. (1974) Unscheduled DNA synthesis in the germ cells of male mice exposed *in vivo* to the chemical mutagen ethyl methanesulphonate. *Proc. Natl. Acad. Sci. USA,* **71,** 4955–4959.

Sega, G.A., Owens, J.G., and Cummings, R.B. (1976) Studies on DNA repair in early spermatid stages of male mice after *in vivo* treatment with methyl-, ethyl-, propyl- and isopropyl methane sulfonate. *Mutat. Res.,* **36,** 193–212.

Setlow, R.B., Regan, J.D., German, J., and Carrier, W.L. (1969) Evidence that cells from Xeroderma pigmentosum do not perform the first step in repair of ultraviolet damage to their DNA. *Proc. Natl. Acad. Sci. USA,* **64,** 1035–1041.

Shapiro, N.I., Petrova, O.N., and Khalizev, A.E. (1968) Induction of gene mutations in mammalian cells *in vitro. Technical Report,* **I.A.E.–1782** (in Russian). Institute of Atomic Energy (Moscow).

Shoemaker, R.C., and Ihrke, C.A. (1983) Effects of the pesticides captan, folpet, guthion and dichlorvos on recombination in maize (*Zea mays* L.). *Environ. Exp. Bot.,* **23,** 45–51.

Thilly, W.G., Deluca, J.G., Furth, E.E., Hoppe, H., Kaden, D.A., Krolewski, J.J., Liber, H.L., Skopek, T.R., Slapikoff, S.A., Tizard, R.J., and Penman, B.W. (1980) Gene-locus mutation assays in diploid human lymphoblast lines. In *Chemical Mutagens* (see de Serres and Hollaender in Gen. Refs.), Vol. 6, pp. 331–364.

Topharn, J.C. (1983) Chemically induced changes in sperm in animals and humans. In *Chemical Mutagens* (see de Serres in Gen. Refs.), Vol. 8, pp. 201–234.

Underbrink, A.G., Schairer, L.A., and Sparrow, A.H. (1973) *Tradescantia* stamen hairs: A radiobiological test system applicable to chemical mutagenesis. In *Chemical Mutagens* (see Hollaender in Gen. Refs.), Vol. 3, pp. 171–207.

Wyrobek, A.J., and Bruce, W.R. (1978) The induction of sperm-shape abnormalities in mice and humans. In *Chemical Mutagens* (see Hollaender and de Serres in Gen. Refs.), Vol. 5, pp. 257–285.

Zbinden, G. (1980) Unscheduled DNA synthesis in the testis, a secondary test for the evaluation of chemical mutagens. *Arch. Toxicol.,* **46,** 139–149.

References to Chapter 2

Adler, I.D. (1970) Cytogenetic analysis of ascites tumour cells of mice in mutation research. In *Chemical Mutagenesis in Mammals and Man* (see Vogel and Röhrborn in Gen. Refs.), pp. 251–259.

Allen, J.W., and Latt, S.A. (1976) Analysis of sister-chromatid exchange formation *in vivo* in mouse spermatogonia as a new test-system for environmental mutagens. *Nature*, **260,** 449–451.

Bateman, A.J. (1958a) The partition of dominant lethals in the mouse between unimplanted eggs and deciduomata. *Heredity,* **12,** 467–475.

Bateman, A.J. (1958b) The two classes of dominant lethal in the mouse. X Int. Congr. Genet. (Montreal), **2,** 14 (Abstract).

Beatty, R.A. (1977) F-bodies as Y-chromosome markers in mature sperm heads: A quantitative approach. *Cytogenet. Cell Genet.,* **18,** 33–49.

Bender, M.A., and Chu, E.H.Y. (1963) In *Evolutionary and Genetic Biology of Primates* (ed. J. Buettner-Janusch), Vol. 1, Academic Press (New York and London).

Bloom, S.E., and Hsu, T.C. (1975) Differential fluorescence of sister-chromatid in chicken embryos exposed to 5-bromodeoxyuridine. *Chromosoma,* **51,** 261–267.

Bobrow, M., and Ejiwunmi, A. (1978) A possible primate model for the study of spontaneous non-disjunction. *XIV Int. Congr. Genet. (Moscow),* **1,** 310 (Abstract).

Brewen, J.G., and Payne, H.S. (1976) Studies on chemically induced dominant lethality. II. Cytogenic studies of MMS-induced dominant lethality in maturing dictyate mouse oocytes. *Mutat. Res.,* **37**, 77–82.

Brewen, J.G., and Payne, H.S. (1978) Studies on chemically induced dominant lethality. III. Cytogenetic analysis of TEM-effects on maturing dicytate mouse oocytes. *Mutat. Res.,* **50,** 85–92.

Brosseau, G.E., Nicoletti, B., Grell, E.H., and Lindsley, D.L. (1961) Production of altered Y-chromosomes bearing specific sections of the X-chromosome in *Drosophila. Genetics,* **46,** 339–346.

Caine, A., and Lyon, M.F., (1977) The induction of chromosome aberrations in mouse dictyate oocytes by X-rays and chemical mutagens. *Mutat. Res.,* **45,** 325–331.

Cattanach, B.M. (1971) Specific locus mutation in mice. In *Chemical Mutagens* (see Hollaender in Gen. Refs.), Vol. 2, pp. 535–539.

Chu, E.H.Y., and Bender, M.A. (1964) Cytogenetics and evolution in primates. *Ann. N.Y. Acad. Sci.,* **102,** 253–266.

Chu, E.H.Y., and Monesi, V. (1960) Analysis of X-ray induced chromosome aberrations in mouse somatic cells *in vitro. Genetics,* **45,** 981 (Abstract).

Ehling, U.H. (1970) The multiple loci method. In *Chemical Mutagenesis in Mammals and Man* (see Vogel and Röhrborn in Gen. Refs.), pp. 156–161.

Ehling, U.H. (1978) Specific-locus mutations in mice. In *Chemical Mutagens* (see Hollaender in Gen. Refs.), Vol. 5, pp. 233–256.

Ehrenberg, L. (1971) Higher plants. In *Chemical Mutagens* (see Hollaender in Gen. Refs.), Vol. 2, pp. 365–386.

Evans, H.J. (1962) Chromosome aberrations induced by ionizing radiations. *Int. Rev. Cytol.,* **13,** 221–321.

Evans, H.J. (1976) Cytological methods for detecting chemical mutagens. In *Chemical Mutagens* (see Hollaender in Gen. Refs.), Vol. 4, pp. 1–29.

Fahrig, R. (1978) The mammalian spot test: A sensitive *in vivo* method for the detection of genetic alterations in somatic cells of mice. In *Chemical Mutagens* (see Hollaender and de Serres in Gen. Refs.) Vol. 5, pp. 151–176.

Giles, N. (1954) Radiation-induced chromosome aberrations in *Tradescantia.* In *Radiation Biology* (see Hollaender in Gen. Refs.), Vol. 1, pp. 713–761.

Gustafsson, Å. (1940) The mutation system of the chlorophyll apparatus. *Lunds Univ. Årsskr. N.F., 2,* **36,** 1–40.

Hansmann, I., and Probek, H.D. (1979) Detection of non-disjunction in mammals. *Environ. Health Perspect.,* **31,** 161–168.

Harnden, D.G. (1960) A human skin culture technique used for cytological examinations. *Br. J. Exp. Pathol.,* **41,** 31–37.

Hirschhorn, K. (1965) Method for studying lymphocyte interaction and other immunologic and cytogenetic studies of human lymphocytes. In *Histocompatibility Testing*, pp. 177–178, National Academy of Science, National Research Council.

Jagiello, G. (1965) A method for meiotic preparations of mammalian ova. *Cytogenetics,* **4,** 245–250.

Jenssen, D., and Ramel, C. (1980) The micronucleus test as a part of a short-term mutagenicity test program for the prediction of carcinogenicity evaluated by 143 agents tested. *Mutat. Res.,* **75,** 191–202.

Kaufmann, B. (1954) Chromosome aberrations induced in animal cells by ionizing radiations. In *Radiation Biology* (see Hollaender in Gen. Refs.), Vol. 1, pp. 627–711.

Klose, J. (1977) The protein-mapping-method employed to test for chemically induced point mutations in mice. *Arch. Toxicol.,* **38,** 53–60.

Krüger, J. (1970) Statistical methods in mutation research. In *Chemical Mutagenesis in*

Mammals and Man (see Vogel and Röhrborn in Gen. Refs.), pp. 460–502.

Latt, S.A., and Allen, J.W. (1977) *In vitro* and *in vivo* analysis of sister-chromatid-exchange formation. In *Handbook of Mutagenicity Test Procedures* (see Kilbey *et al.* in Gen. Refs.), pp. 275–291. (1977).

Legator, J.S., Truong, L., and Connor, T.H. (1978) Analysis of body fluids including alkylation of macromolecules for detection of mutagenic agents. In *Chemical Mutagens* (see Hollaender and de Serres in Gen. Refs.), Vol. 5, pp. 1–23.

Lindsley, D.L., and Grell, E.H. (1967) Genetic variations of *Drosophila melanogaster. Carnegie Inst. Washington Publ.,* **627.**

Lyon, M.F., and Morris, T. (1966) Mutation rates at a new set of specific loci in the mouse. *Genet. Res.,* **7,** 12–17.

Lyon, M.F., and Morris, T. (1969) Gene and chromosome mutation after large fractionated and unfractionated radiation doses to mouse spermatogonia. *Mutat. Res.,* **8,** 191–198.

MacKey J. (1967) Physical and chemical mutagenesis in relations to ploidy level. Induzierte Mutationen und ihre Nutzung. Erwin-Baur Gedächtnisvorl. IV Gatersleben, 1966. *Abh. Dtsch. Akad. Wiss. Berlin Kl. Med.,* **2,** 185–197.

Malling, H.V., and Valcovic, L.R. (1977) A biochemical specific locus mutation system in mice. *Arch. Toxicol.,* **38,** 45–51.

Moutschen, J. (1969) Mutagenesis with methyl methanesulfonate in mouse. *Mutat. Res.,* **8,** 581–588.

Moutschen, J. (1970) Sur la cinétique des aberrations de la structure chromosomique dues aux radiations ionisantes et aux agents d'alkylation. *Bull. Soc. Bot. Fr.,* **117,** 341–352.

Muller, H.J., and Oster, I.I. (1963) Some mutational techniques in *Drosophila* In *Methodology in Basic Genetics* (see Burdette in Gen. Refs.) pp. 249–278.

Nilan, R.A., and Vig, B.K. (1976) Plant test systems for detection of chemical mutagens. In *Chemical Mutagens* (see Hollaender in Gen. Refs.), vol. 4, pp. 143–170.

Röbbelen, G. (1964) Futile attempt of mutation with some base analogues and antimetabolites. *Arabidopsis Inf. Serv.,* **1,** 20–21.

Röhrborn, G. (1970) The dominant lethals: method and cytogenic examination of early cleavage stages. In *Chemical Mutagens in Mammals and Man* (see Vogel and Röhrborn in Gen. Refs.), pp. 148–155).

Russel, L.B. (1976) Numerical sex-chromosome anomalies in mammals: Their spontaneous occurrence and use in mutagenesis studies. In *Chemical Mutagens* (see Hollaender in Gen. Refs.), Vol. 4, pp. 55–91.

Russel, L.B., and Major, M.M. (1957) Radiation-induced presumed somatic mutations in the house mouse. *Genetics,* **42,** 161–175.

Russel, L.B., and Saylors, C.L. (1963) The relative sensitivity of various germ-cells stages of the mouse to raidation-induced nondisjunction, chromosome losses and deficiencies. In *Repair from Genetic Radiation Damage and Differential Radiosensitivity in Germ Cells* (ed. F. Sobels), pp. 313–342. Pergamon Press (Oxford, London, New York and Paris).

Russel, L.B., Russel, W., Popp, R.A., Vaughan, C., and Jacobson, K. (1976) Radiation-induced mutations at mouse hemoglobin loci. *Proc. Natl. Acad. Sci. USA,* **73,** 2843–2846.

Russel, L.B., Selby, P.B., von Halle, E., Sheridan, W., and Valcovic, L. (1981a) The mouse specific-locus test with agents other than radiations. *Mutat. Res.,* **86,** 329–354.

Russel, L.B., Selby, P.B., von Halle, E., Sheridan, W., and Valcovic, L. (1981b) Use of the mouse spot test in chemical mutagenesis. *Mutat. Res.,* **86,** 355–379.

Russel, W.L. (1951) X-Ray induced mutations in mice. *Cold Spring Harbor Symp. Quant. Biol.,* **16,** 327–336.

Russel, W. (1965) The nature of the dose-rate effect of radiation on mutation in mice. *Genetics* **40,** (*Suppl.1) 128—140.*

Russel, W.L. Russel, L.B., and Kimball, A.W. (1954) The relative effectiveness of neutrons from a nuclear detonation and from a cyclotron in inducing dominant lethals in the mouse. *Am. Nat.*, **88**, 269–286.

Schmid, (1976) The micronucleus test for cytogenetic analysis. In *Chemical Mutagens* (see Hollaender and de Serres in Gen. Refs.), Vol. 4, pp, 31–53.

Smith, R.H., and von Borstel, R.C. (1971) Inducing mutations with chemicals in *Habrobracon*. In *Chemical Mutagens* (see Hollaender in Gen. Refs.), Vol. 2, pp. 445–460.

Stadler, L.J. (1928) Genetic effects of X-rays in maize. *Proc. Natl. Acad. Sci. USA,* **14,** 69–75.

Tarkowski, A.K. (1966) An air-drying method for chromosome preparations from mouse eggs. *Cytogenetics,* **5,** 394–400.

Taylor, J.H. (1958) Sister chromatid exchanges in tritium-labelled chromosomes. *Genetics,* **43,** 515–529.

Telfer, J.D. (1954) An improved technique for dominant lethal studies in *Drosophila. Am. Nat.,* **88,** 117–118.

Tjio, J.H., and Whang, J. (1962) Chromosome preparations of bone marrow cells without prior *in vitro* culture or *in vivo* colchicine administration. *Stain Technol.,* **37,** 17–20.

Vogel, W., and Bauknecht, T. (1976) Differential chromatid staining by *in vivo* treatment as a mutagenicity test system. *Nature,* **260,** 448–449.

Whiting, A.R. (1961) Genetics of *Habrobracon. Adv. Genet.,* **10,** 295–348.

References to Chapter 3

Abrahamson, S., Würgler, F.E., Dejongh, C., and Unger Meyer, H.U. (1980) How many loci on the X-chromosome of *Drosophila melanogaster* can mutate to recessive lethals? *Environ. Mutagenesis,* **2**, 447–453.

Bobrow, M., and Ejiwunmi, A. (1978) A possible primate model for the study of spontaneous non-disjunction. XIV Int. Congr. Genet. (Moscow), **1,** 310 (Abstract).

Brink, R.A. (1958) Mutable loci and development of the organism. Symposium on genetic approaches to somatic cell variations. *Cell. Comp. Physiol.,* **52** (*Suppl.*), 169–195.

Ehrenberg, L. (1977) Aspects of statistical inference in testing for genetic toxicity. In *Handbook of Mutagenicity Test Procedures* (see Kilbey, *et al.* in Gen. Refs.), pp. 419–459.

Ehrenberg, L., and Eriksson, G. (1966) The dose dependence of mutation rates in the rad range, in the light of experiments with higher plants. *Acta Radiol. (Suppl.),* **254,** 73–81.

Ehrenberg, L., Hiesche, K.D., Osterman-Golkar, S., and Wennberg, I. (1974) Evaluation of genetic risks of alkylating agents: Tissue doses in the mouse from air contaminated with ethylene oxide. *Mutat. Res.,* **24,** 83–103.

Evans, H.J. (1977) Molecular mechanisms in the induction of chromosome aberrations. In *Progress in Genetic Toxicology* (see Scott, Bridges and Sobels in Gen. Refs.), pp. 57–74.

Evans, H.J., (1982) Genetic factors in the response to environmental mutagens. In *Environmental Mutagens and Carcinogens* (see Sugimura, Kondo and Takebe in Gen. Refs.), pp. 599–601.

Fraser, F.C. (1981) The genetics of common familia disorders — major genes or multi factorial? *Can. J. Genet.*, **23,** 1–8.

Haynes, R.H., and Eckhardt, F. (1980) Mathematical analysis of mutation induction kinetics. In *Chemical Mutagens* (see de Serres and Hollaender in Gen. Refs.), vol. 6, pp. 271–304.

Howard, A., and Haigh, M.V. (1968) Chloroplast aberrations in irradiated fern spores. *Mutat. Res.,* **6,** 263–280.

Kastenbaum, M.A., and Bowman, K.O. (1970) Tables for determining the significance of mutation frequencies. *Mutat. Res.,* **9,** 527–549.

Klekowski, E. Jr. Detection of mutational damage in fern populations; an *in situ* bioassay for mutagens in aquatic ecosystems. In *Chemical Mutagens* (see Hollaender and de Serres in Gen. Refs.), Vol. 5, pp. 79–99.

Kratochvilova, J. (1981) Dominant cataract mutations detected in offspring of gamma irradiated male mice. *J. Hered.,* **72,** 302–307.

Kratochvilova, J., and Ehling, U. (1979) Dominant cataract mutations induced by gamma irradiation of male mice. *Mutat. Res.,* **63,**, 221–223.

Kruger, J. (1971) Statistical methods in mutation research (Appendix). In *Chemical Mutagenesis in Mammals and Man* (see Vogel and Röhrborn in Gen. Refs.), pp. 460–502.

Malling, H. (1981) Perspectives in mutagenesis. *Environ. Mutagenesis,* **3,** 103–108.

Marin, G., and Prescott, D.M. (1964) The frequency of sister chromatid exchanges following exposure to varying doses of H3-thymidine or X-rays. *J. Cell Biol.,* **21,** 159–167.

Moutschen, J. (1962) Effets génétiques retardés du Myleran chez *Osmunda regalis* L. *Lejeunia (Nouv. Sér.),* **11,** 1–15.

Moutschen, J., and Colizzi, A. (1975) Absence of acrosome: an efficient tool in mammalian mutation research. *Mutat. Res.,* **30,** 267–272.

Moutschen, J., and Moutschen-Dahmen, M. (1958) L'action du Myleran (di-méthane-sulfonyloxybutane) sur les chromosomes chez *Hordeum sativum* et chez *Vicia faba. Hereditas,* **44,** 415–446.

Moutschen, J., and Moutschen-Dahmen, M. (1971) Use of *Chara* antheridial chromosomes for estimating water pollution. *First Ann. Meet. Eur. Environ. Mutagen Soc.,* (Noorwijkerhout, The Netherlands) (Abstract).

Ramel, C. (1983) Polygenic effects and genetic changes affecting quantitative traits. (ICPEMC Publ. No. 8.), *Mutat. Res.,* **114**, 107–116.

Russel, W.L. (1951) X-ray-induced mutations in mice. *Cold Spring Harbor Symposia Quant. Biol.,* **16,** 327–336.

Sparrow, A.H., Underbrink, A.G., and Rossi, H.H. (1972) Mutations induced in *Tradescantia* by small doses of X-rays and neutrons: Analysis of dose–response curves. *Science,* **176,** 916–918.

Sulovska, K., Lindgren, D., Eriksson, G., and Ehrenberg, L. (1969) The mutagenic effect of low concentrations of ethylene oxide in air. *Hereditas,* **62**, 264–266.

Wolff, S., (1977) Sister chromatid exchanges. *Annu. Rev. Genet.,* **11,** 183–201.

Würgler, F.L., Graf, U., and Berchtold, W. (1975) Statistical problems connected with the sex-linked recessive lethal test in *Drosophila melanogaster.* I. The use of the Kastenbaum – Bowman test. *Arch. Genet.,* **48,** 158–178.

References to Chapter 4

Adler, I.D. (1970) The problem of caffeine mutagenicity. In *Chemical Mutagenesis in Mammals and Man* (see Vogel and Röhrborn in Gen. refs.), pp, 383–403.

Altenburg, E., and Browning, L.S. (1964) The rate of gonadal mosaicism for lethals in late broods of *Drosophila* as compared with early when induced by X-rays, azaserine and quinacrine mustard. *Genetics,* **50,** 232.

Anderson, K.J. (1979) Platinum II complexes generate frame-shift mutations in test strains of *Salmonella typhimurium. Mutat. Res.,* **67,** 209–214.

Andrew, L.E. (1959) The mutagenic activity of caffeine in *Drosophila. Am. Nat.,* **93,** 135–138.

Auerbach, C. (1949) Chemical mutagenesis. *Biol. Rev. Cambridge Philos. Soc.*, **24,** 355–391.

Auerbach, C. (1952) Mutation tests on *Drosophila melanogaster* with aqueous solutions of formaldehyde. *Am. Nat.*, **86,** 330–332.

Auerbach, C., and Robson, J.M. (1944) Production of mutations by allyl isothiocyanate. *Nature,* **154,** 81.

Auerbach, C., and Robson, J.M. (1947) Tests of chemical substances for mutagenic action. *Proc. R. Soc. Edinburgh Sect. B,* **62,** 284–291.

Auerbach, C., Robson, J.M., and Carr, J.G. (1947) The chemical production of mutations. *Science*, **105,** 243–247.

Auerbach, C., Moutschen-Dahmen, M., and Moutschen, J. (1977) Genetic and cytogenetical effects of formaldehyde and related compounds. *Mutat. Res.,* **39,** 317–362.

Bacchetti, S., and Graham, F.L. (1977) Transfer of the gene for thymidine kinase to thymidine kinase-deficient human cells by purified herpes simplex viral DNA. *Proc. Natl. Acad. Sci. USA,* **74,** 1590–1594.

Bacchetti, S., and Graham, F.L. (1978) *IARC Sci. Publ.*, **24**, 495–499.

Baden, J.M., and Simmon, V. (1980) Mutagenic effects of inhalational anesthetics. *Mutat. Res.*, **75,** 169–189.

Bartsch, H.D. (1970) Virus-induced chromosomal aberrations in mammals and man. In *Chemical Mutagenesis in Mammals and Man* (see Vogel and Röhrborn in Gen. Refs.), pp. 420–432.

Batzinger, R.P., Buedinge, Reddy, B.S., and Weisburger, J.H., (1978) Formation of a mutagenic drug metabolite by intestinal microorganism. *Cancer Res.*, **38,** 608–612.

Beck, D.J., and Fisch, J.E. (1980) Mutagenicity of platinum coordination complexes in *Salmonella typhimurium. Mutat. Res.,* **77,** 45–54.

Bender, L., and Sankar, S. (1968) Chromosome damage not found in leukocytes of children treated with LSD-25. *Science,* **159,** 749.

Biesele, J.J. (1958) Chemically induced imitations of mitotic anomalies common to cancer cells. *Ann. N.Y. Acad. Sci.,* **71,** 1054–1067.

Bishun, N., Mills, J., and Williams, D. (1973) Chromosomes and 'the pill'. *Mutat. Res.,* **21**, 186.

Bishun, N., Smith, N., Williams, D., and Mills, J. (1976) Cytological effects of the oral contraceptive. *Mutat. Res.,* **39,** 97–110.

Blair, D., Hoadleye, C., and Hutson, D. (1975) The distribution of dichlorvos in the tissues of mammals after its inhalation or intravenous administration. *Toxicol. Appl. Pharmacol.,* **31,** 243–253.

Bornstein, R.S., Hungerford, D.K., Haller, G., Engström, P.F., and Yarbro, J.M. (1971) Cytogenetic effects of bleomycin therapy in man. *Cancer Res.,* **31**, 2004–2007.

Brown, J.P. (1980) Flavonoids, anthraquinones and related compounds. *Mutat. Res.*, **75,** 243–277.

Brown, R.L., and Crossen, P.E. (1976) Increased incidence of sister chromatid exchanges in Rauscher leukaemia virus infected mouse embryo fibroblasts. *Exp. Cell Res.,* **103**, 418–420.

Browning, L.S. (1968) Lysergic acid diethylamide: mutagenic effects in *Drosophila. Science,* **161,** 1022–1023.

Camara, A., and Angulo-Carpio, D. (1949) Influencia de la morfina sobre la meiosis de *Triticum. Genet. Iber.*, **1,** 13–26.

Carr, D.H. (1967) Chromosomes after oral contraceptives. *Lancet*, **ii,** 830–831.

Cattanach, B.M. (1962) Genetic effects of caffeine in mice. *Z. Vererbungsl.,* **93,** 215–219.

Cattanach, B.M. (1976) The mutagenicity of cyclamates and their metabolites. *Mutat. Res.,* **39,** 1–28.

Clark, A.M., and Clark, E.G. (1968) The genetic effects of caffeine in *Drosophila melanogaster*. *Mutat. Res.,* **6,** 227–234.

Clemmesen, J. (1981) Epidemiological studies into the possible carcinogenicity of hair dyes. *Mutat. Res.,* **87,** 65–79.

Cohen, M.M., and Shaw, M.W. (1964) Effects of mitomycin C on human chromosomes. *J. Cell Biol.,* **23,** 386–395.

Cohen, M.M., Shaw, M.W., and Craig, A.P. (1963) The effects of streptonigrin on cultured human leukocytes. *Proc. Natl. Acad. Sci. USA,* **50,** 16–24.

Cohen, M.M., Marinello, M.J., and Beck, N. (1967a) Chromosomal damage in human leukocytes induced by lysergic acid diethylamide. *Science,* **155,** 1417–1419.

Cohen, M.M., Hirschhorn, K., and Forsch, W.A. (1967b) *In vivo* and *in vitro* chromosomal damage induced by LSD-25 *N. Engl. J. Med.,* **277,** 1043–1049.

Combes, R.D., and Haveland-Smith, R.B. (1982) A review of the genotoxicity of food, drug and cosmetic colours and other azo, triphenylmethane and xanthine dyes. *Mutat. Res.,* **98,** 101–248.

Commoner, B., Vithayathic, A.J., Dolara, P., Nair, S., Madyastha, P., and Cuca, G.C. (1978) Formation of mutagens in beef and beef extract during cooking. *Science,* **201,** 913–916.

Davidson, D. (1965) Chromosomal breakage and reunion: action of azaserine and X-rays. *Z. Vererbl.,* **96,** 217–227.

Degraeve, N. (1978) Genetic and related effects of *Vinca rosea* alkaloids *Mutat. Res.,* **55,** 31–42.

Degraeve, N., Moutschen, J., Moutschen-Dahmen, M., Houbrechts, N., and Colizzi, A. (1976) A propos des risques d'un insecticide: le carbaryl utilisé seul et en combinaison avec les nitrites. *Bull. Soc. R. Sci. Liège,* **45,** 46–57.

Delone, N.L. (1958) *Dokl. Akad. Nauk SSSR,* **119,** 800; *Chem. Abst.,* **52,** 15660 (1958).

Delone, N.L. (1958) *Biofizika*, 3, 717; *Chem. Abst.* **53,** 4448 (1959).

Demerec, M., Wallace, B., and Wither, E.M. (1948) The gene. *Carnegie Inst. Washington Yearb.,* **47,** 169–176.

Demerec, M., Bertani, G., and Flint, J., (1951) A survey of chemicals for mutagenic action on *Escherichia coli. Am. Nat.,* **85,** 119–136.

Draper, M.H., and Griffin, J.P. (1980) Draft guidelines on mutagenicity testing of new drugs issues by the CPMP. A four test screen. *Arch. Toxicol.,* **46,** 9–19.

Eberle, P., and Leuner, H. (1970) Chromosomendefekte bei Psilocybin-Patienten. *Humangenetik,* **9,** 281–285.

Ehrenberg, L., and Hallström, T. (1967) Haematologic studies on persons occupationally exposed to ethylene oxide. In *Radiosterilization of Medical Products*. International Atomic Energy Agency (Vienna), pp. 327–334.

Ehrenberg, L., and Hussain, S. (1981) Genetic toxicity of some important epoxides. *Mutat. Res.,* **86,** 1–113.

Ehrenberg, L., Gustafsson, Å., and von Wettstein, D. (1956) Studies on the mutation process in plants-regularities and intentional control. *Conference on Chromosomes, Wageningen,* (Netherlands), pp. 131–159.

Ehrenberg, L., Hiesche, K.D., Osterman-Golkar, S., and Wennberg, I. (1974) Evaluation of genetic risks of alkylating agents: tissue doses in the mouse from air contaminated with ethylene oxide. *Mutat. Res.,* **24,** 83–103.

El-Alfi, O.S., Smith, P.M., and Biesele, J.J. (1965) Chromosomal breaks in human leucocyte cultures induced by an agent in the plasma of infectious hepatitis patients. *Hereditas,* **52,** 285–294.

Elespuru, R., Lijinksy, W., and Setlow, J. (1974) Nitroso-carbaryl as a potent mutagen of environmental significance. *Nature,* (London), **247,** 386–387.

Epstein, S. (1970) The failure of caffeine to induce mutagenic effects or to synergize the effects of known mutagens in mice. In *Chemical Mutagenesis in Mammals and Man* (see Vogel and Röhrborn in Gen. Refs.), pp. 404–419.

Evans, I.A. (1968) The radiomimetic nature of bracken toxin. *Cancer Res.,* **28,** 2252–2261.

Evans, I.A., and Mason, J. (1965) Veterinary science. Carcinogenic activity of bracken. *Nature,* **208,** 913–914.

Falek, A., Jordan, R.B., King, B.J., Arnold, P.J. and Skelton, W.D. (1972) Human chromosomes and opiates. *Arch. Gen. Psychiatry,* **27,** 511–515.

Fogh, J., and Fogh, H. (1967) Irreversibility of major chromosome change in mycoplasma modified line of FL human amnion cells. *Proc. Soc. Exp. Biol. Med.,* **26,** 67–74.

Freese, E., Sklarow, S., and Bautz Freese, E. (1968) DNA damage caused by antidepressant hydrazines and related drugs. *Mutat. Res.,* **5,** 343–348.

Fries, N. (1948) Viability and resistance of spontaneous mutations in *Ophiostoma,* representing different degrees of heterotrophy. *Physiol. Planta.* **1,** 330–341.

Fries, N., and Kihlman, B. (1948) Fungal mutations obtained with methylxanthines. *Nature,* **162,** 573–574.

Funès-Cravioto, F., Lambert, B., Lindstein, J., Ehrenberg, L., Natarajan, A.T. and Osterman-Golkar, S. (1975) Chromosome aberrations in workers exposed to vinyl chloride. *Lancet,* **i**, 459.

Gabridge, M.G., Oswald, E.J., and Legator, M.S. (1969) The role of selection in the host-mediated assay for mutagenicity. *Mutat. Res.,* **7,** 117–119.

Gilmour, D.G., Bloom A.D., Lele K.P., Robbins, E.S., and Maximilian C. (1971) Chromosomal aberrations in users of psychoactive drugs. *Arch. Gen. Psychiat.,* **24,** 268–272.

Gilot-Delhalle, J., and Moutschen, J. (1972) On the origin of ethyl methane sulfonate induced sterility in *Nigella damascena. Radiat. Bot.,* **12,** 381–384.

Gilot, J., Delhalle, J., Colizzi, A., Moutschen, J., and Moutschen-Dahmen, M. (1983) Mutagenicity of some organophosphorus compounds at the *ade 6* locus of *Schizosaccharomyces pombe. Mutat. Res.,* **117,** 139–148.

Grace, D., Carlson, E.A., and Goodman, P. (1968) *Drosophila melanogaster* treated with LSD: Absence of mutation and chromosomic breakage. *Science,* **161,** 694–696.

Gustafsson, Å., and McKey, J. (1948) The genetical effects of mustard gas substances and neutrons. *Hereditas,* **34,** 371–386.

Halkka, O. (1967) Chromosome breakage associated with infection. I. Phase contrast microscopy. *Hereditas,* **58,** 248–252.

Hampar, G., and Elisson, S.A. (1961) Chromosomal aberrations induced by an animal virus. *Nature,* **192,** 145–147.

Harnden, D.G. (1964) Cytogenetic studies on patients with virus infections and subjects vaccinated against yellow fever. *Am. J. Hum. Genet.,* **16,** 201–213.

Haveland-Smith, R.B. (1981) Evaluation of the genotoxicity of some natural colours using bacterial assays. *Mutat. Res.,* **91,** 285–290.

Ignoffo, C.M. (1968) Virus-living insecticides. *Curr. Top. Microbiol.,* **42,** 129–167.

Irwin, S., and Egozcue, J. (1967) Chromosomal abnormalities in leukocytes from LSD-25 users. *Science,* **157,** 313–314.

Jacobs, N.F., Neu, R.L., and Gardner, L.I. (1969) Phleomycin-induced mitotic inhibition and chromosomal abnormalities in cultured human leukocytes. *Mutat. Res.,* **7,** 251–253.

Jagiello, G.M. (1967) Streptonigrin: Effect on the first meiotic metaphase of the mouse egg. *Science,* **157,** 453–454.

Jagiello, G.M. (1968) Action of phleomycin on the meiosis of the mouse ovum. *Mutat. Res.,* **6,** 289–295.

Jarvik, L.F., and Kato, T. (1968) Is lysergide a teratogen? *Lancet,* **i,** 250.

Kaplan, W.D. (1948) Formaldehyde as a mutagen in *Drosophila. Science,* **108,** 43.

Kaplanis, J.N., Thompson, M.J., Robbins, W.E., and Bryce, M. (1967) Insect hormones: Alpha ecdysone and 20-hydroxyecdysone in bracken fern. *Science,* **157,** 1436–1438.

Kato, R. (1967) Localization of 'spontaneous' and Rous sarcoma virus-induced breakage in specific regions of the chromosomes of the Chinese hamster. *Hereditas,* **58,** 221–247.

Kato, R. (1968) The chromosomes of forty-two primary Rous sarcomas of the chinese hamster. *Hereditas,* **59,** 63–119.

Kaufmann, B.P., and McDonald, M.R. (1957) The nature of the changes effected in chromosomal materials by the chelating agent EDTA. *Proc. Natl. Acad. Sci. USA,* **43,** 262–270.

Khristol-Yubova, N.B. (1961) *Dokl. Akad. Nauk SSSR,* **138,** 681; *Chem. Abstr.,* **55,** 21.396

Kihlman, B.A. (1952) A survey of purine derivatives as inducers of chromosome changes. *Hereditas,* **38,** 115–127.

Kihlman, B.A. (1955) Chromosome breakage in *Allium* by 8-ethoxycaffeine and X-rays. *Expt. Cell Res.,* **8,** 345–368.

Kihlman, B.A. (1964) The production of chromosomal aberrations by streptonigrin in *Vicia faba. Mutat. Res.,* **1,** 54–62.

Kihlman, B.A., and Levan, A. (1949) The cytological effect of caffeine. *Hereditas,* **35,** 109–111.

Kihlman, B.A., and Odmark, G. (1965) Deoxyribonucleic acid synthesis and the production of chromosomal aberrations by streptonigrin, 8-ethoxycaffeine and 1, 3, 7, 9-tetramethyluric acid. *Mutat. Res.,* **2,** 494–505.

Kihlman, B.A., Odmark, G., and Hartley, B. (1967) Studies on the effects of phleomycin on chromosome structure and nucleic acid synthesis in *Vicia faba. Mutat. Res.,* **4,** 783–790.

Kimball, R.F. (1977) The mutagenicity of hydrazine and some of its derivatives. *Mutat. Res.,* **39,** 111–126.

Kramers, P.G.N. (1975) The mutagenicity of saccharin. *Mutat. Res.,* **32**, 81–92.

Kulkarni, R.K., Bartak, D., Ousterhout, D.K., and Leonard, F. (1968) Determination of residual ethylene oxide in catheters by gas–liquid chromatography. *J. Biomed. Mater. Res.,* **2,** 165–171.

Latt, S.A. (1974) Sister chromatid exchanges, indices of human chromosome damage and repair: detection by fluorescence and induction by mitomycin. *Proc. Natl. Acad. Sci. USA,* **71,** 3162–3165.

Legator, M. (1968) *Med. World News,* **9,** 25.

Legator, M., Palmer, K.A., Green, S., and Petersen, K.W. (1969) Cytogenetic studies in rats of cyclohexylamine, a metabolite of cyclamate. *Science,* **165,** 1139–1140.

Lithmer, F., and Pontén, J. (1966) Bovine fibroblasts in long term tissue culture: chromosome studies. *Int. J. Cancer,* **1,** 579–586.

Loprieno, N., Barale, R., Mariani, L., and Zaccaro, L. (1982) Mutagenic studies on the hair dye 2(2′,4′-diaminophenoxy)ethanol with different genetic systems. *Mutat. Res.,* **102,** 331–346.

Loughman, W.D., Sargent, T.W., and Israelstam, D.M. (1967) Leukocytes of humans exposed to lysergic acid diethylamide: Lack of chromosomal damage. *Science,* **158,** 508–510.

Lyon, M.F., Phillips, J.S.R., and Searle, A.G. (1962) A test for mutagenicity of caffeine in mice. *Z. Vererbungsl.,* **93,** 7–13.

Makino, S., and Aya, T. (1968) Cytogenetic studies in leukocyte cultures from patients with some viral diseases and in those infected with Hsv. *Cytologia,* **33,** 370–396.

Marfey, P., and Robinson, E. (1981) Genetic toxicology of hydroxylamines. *Mutat. Res.,* **86,** 155–191.

Matsaniotis, N.K., Kiossoglou, K.A., Maounis, F., and Anagnostakis, D.E. (1966) Chromosomes in infectious hepatitis. *Lancet,* **ii,** 1421.

Matsuoka, A., Hayajhi, M., and Ishidate, M., Jr. (1979) Chromosomal aberration tests on 29 chemicals combined with 59 mix *in vitro. Mutat. Res.,* **66,** 277–290.

Mattingly, E. (1967) Induction of chromosome and chromatid-type aberrations by phleomycin. *Mutat. Res.,* **4,** 51–57.

McDonald, M.R., and Kaufmann, B.P. (1957) Production of mitotic abnormalities by ethylenediaminetetraacetic acid. *Exp. Cell Res.,* **12,** 415–417.

Mella, B., and Lang, D.J. (1967) Leukocytes mitosis: Suppression *in vitro* associated with acute infectious hepatitis. *Science,* **155,** 80–81.

Merz, T. (1961) Effect of mitomycin C on lateral root-tip chromosomes of *Vicia faba. Science,* **133,** 329–330.

Miyamoto, J. (1976) Degradation, metabolism and toxicity of synthetic pyrethroid. *Environ. Health Perspect.,* **14,** 15–28.

Morad, M.J., Jonasson, J., and Lindsten, J. (1973) Distribution of mitomycin C induced breaks on human chromosomes. *Hereditas,* **74,** 273–282.

Morgan, R.W., and Hoffmann, G. (1983) Cycasin and its mutagenic metabolites. *Mutat. Res.,* **114,** 19–58.

Morrison, W.D., Huff, V., Colyer, S.P., Dufrain, R.J., and Littlefield, L.G. (1981) Cytogenetic effects of *cis*-platinum(II) diamminodichloride *in vivo. Environ. Mutagenesis,* **3**, 265–274.

Moutschen, J., (1979) Pesticides: from plants to man. *Ethics and Genetics*, UNESCO, Madrid (1958), 263–275.

Moutschen, J., and Moutschen-Dahmen, M. (1958), Sur l'évolution des lésions causées par la 8-éthoxycaféine chez *Hordeum sativum et chez Vicia faba. Hereditas,* **44,** 415–446.

Moutschen, J., Gilot-Delhalle, J., and Thakare, R.G. (1973a) Modifications by means of an antibiotic of the effect of Co^{60} gamma radiations at the chromosome level. *Kerntechnik*, **15,** 72–74.

Moutschen, J., Moutschen-Dahmen, M., and Deby, C. (1973b) Hazards of prostaglandins for chromosome damage. *Mutat. Res.,* **21**, 42–43.

Moutschen, J., Moutschen-Dahmen, M., and Degraeve, N. (1981) Metrifonate and dichlorvos, Cytogenetic investigations. *Acta Pharmacol. Toxicol.*, 49 (*Suppl.* V), 29–39.

Moutschen, J., Moutschen-Dahmen, M., and Degraeve, N. (1984) Mutagenicity, carcinogenicity and teratogenicity of insecticides. In *Mutagenicity, Carcinogenicity and Teratogenicity of Industrial Pollutants* (see Kirsch-Volders in Gen. Refs.), pp. 127–203.

Moutschen, J., Moutschen-Dahmen, M., and Gilot-Dehalle, J. (1969) Les processus de réparation des lésions de la classe chromosomique induites par les rayons γ du Co^{60} chez *Nigella damascena* L. *Med. Nucl. Radiobiol. Lat.*, **12**, 17–32.

Moutschen, J., Moutschen-Dahmen, M., Degraeve, N., Houbrechts, N., and Colizzi, A. (1975) Genetical hazards of aldehydes from mouse experiments. *Mutat. Res.,* **29**, 205.

Moutschen, J., Moutschen-Dahmen, M., Houbrechts, N., and Colizzi, A. (1976) Cytotoxicité et mutagénicité de deux aldéhydes: crotonaldéhyde et butyraldéhyde chez la souris. *Bull. Soc. R. Sci. Liège,* **45,** 58–72.

Mukherjee, R. (1965) Mutagenic action of mitomycin C on *Drosophila melanogaster. Genetics.* **51,** 947–951.

Nagao, M., Honda, M., Seino, Y., Yahagi, T., and Sugimura, T. (1977) Mutagenicities of smoke condensates and the charred surface of fish and meat. *Cancer Lett.*, **2,** 221–226.

Natarajan, A.T., and Ahnström, G. (1968) Cytogenetical effects of inorganic pyrophosphate and 5-fluorodeoxyuridine. *Hereditas,* **59,** 229–241.

Nichols, W.W. (1963) Relationships of viruses, chromosomes and carcinogenesis. *Hereditas,* **50,** 53–80.

Nichols, W.W. (1982) Virus induced cellular genetic changes. In *Environmental*

Mutagens and Carcinogens (see Sugimura, *et al.* in Gen. Refs.), pp. 443–454.

Nichols, W.W., Bradt, C.I., Toji, L.H., Godley, M., and Segawa, M. (1978) Induction of sister chromatid exchanges by transformation with Simian Virus 40. *Cancer Res.,* **38**, 960–964.

Nielsen, J., Friedrich, U., and Tsuboi, T. (1968) Chromosome abnormalities and psychotropic drugs. *Nature,* **218**, 488–489.

Nowell, P.C. (1964) Mitotic inhibition and chromosome damage by mitomycin in human leukocyte cultures. *Expl. Cell Res.,* **33,** 445–449.

Oehlkers, F. (1953) Chromosome breaks influenced by chemicals. Symposium on chromosome breakage. *Heridity*, **6** (*Suppl.*), 95–105.

Ohama, K., and Kadotani, T. (1970) Cytologic effects of bleomycin on cultured human leukocytes. *Jp. J. Hum. Gen.*, **14,** 293–297.

Ostertag, W. (1966) Koffein und Theophyllinmutagenese bei Zell und Leukozytenkulturen des Menschen. *Mutat. Res.,* **3,** 249–267.

Ostertag, W., Duisberg, E., and Stürmann, M. (1965) The mutagenic activity of caffeine in man. *Mutat. Res.,* **2,** 293–296.

Ostertag, W., and Haake, J. (1966) The mutagenicity in *Drosophilia melanogaster* of caffeine and other compounds which produce chromosome breakage in human cells in culture. *Z. Vererbungbl.,* **98,** 299–308.

Owen, J.J.T., Moore, M.A.S., and Biggs, P.M. (1966) Chromosome studies in Marek's disease. *J. Natl. Cancer Inst.,* **37,** 199.

Parádi, E. (1981) Mutagenicity of some contraceptive drugs in *Drosophila melanogaster. Mutat. Res.,* **88,** 175–178.

Peer, R.L., and Litz, D.A. (1981) The mutagenic effect of cis-diammine dichloroplatinum (II) and its degradation products in the Ames microbial assay. *Environ. Mutagenesis,* **3,** 555–563.

Perry, S., and Evans, H.H., (1975) Cytological detection of mutagen-carcinogen exposure by sister-chromatid exchanges. *Nature,* **258,** 121–125.

Poland, A., and Glover, E. (1974) Comparison of 2,3,7,8-tetrachlorodibenzo-*p*-dioxin, a potent inducer of aryl hydrocarbon hydroxylase, with 3-methylcholanthrene. *Mol. Pharmacol.,* **10,** 349–359.

Puck, T.T. (1964) Phasing mitotic delay and chromosomal aberrations in mammalian cells. *Science,* **144,** 565–566.

Ragelis, E.P., Fischer, B.S., Klimeck, B.A., and Johnson, C. (1968) Isolation and determination of chlorohydrins in foods fumigated with ethylene oxide or with propylene oxide. *J. Ass. Off. Anal. Chem.,* **51,** 709–715.

Rannug, U. (1980) Genotoxic effects of 1, 2-dibromoethane and 1,2-dichloroethane. *Mutat. Res.,* **76,** 269–295.

Rapoport, I.A. (1946) Carbonyl compounds and the chemical mechanism of mutation. *C.R. Akad. Sci. URSS,* **54,** 65–67.

Rapoport, I.A. (1948) Mutations under the influence of unsaturated aldehydes. *Dokl. Akad. Nauk SSSR,* **61,** 713–715.

Sanders, H.J. (1969) Chemical mutagens. An expanding roster of suspects. *Chem. Eng. News,* **47,** 54–68.

Sax, K., and Sax, H.J. (1968) Possible mutagenic hazards of some food additives, beverages and insecticides. *Jp. J. Genet.,* **43,** 89–94.

Scheibe, A. (1959) Mutationauslösung durch Chemikalien bei Gerste und Weizen. *Deuxième Congrès de l'Eucarpia,* Cologne.

Sentein, P. (1962) L'action du sulfate d'amphétamine et de substances voisines sur les mitoses de segmentation. *Acta Anat.,* **49,** 297–327.

Sharma, K., and Sharma, A. (1962) A study of the importance of nucleic acids in controlling chromosome breaks induced by different compounds. *Nucleus,* **5,** 127–136.

Shaw, M.W., and Cohen, M.M. (1965) Chromosome exchanges in human leukocytes induced by mitomycin C. *Genetics,* **51**, 181–190.

Smith, D.W.E. (1966) Mutagenicity of cycasin aglycone (methylazoxymethanol) a naturally occurring carcinogen. *Science,* **152,** 1273–1274.

Smith, R.H. (1969) Induction of mutations in *Habrobracon* sperm with mitomycin C. *Mutat. Res.,* **7,** 231–234.

Sparkes, R.S., Melynk, J., and Bozzetti, L.P. (1968) Chromosomal effect *in vitro* of exposure to lysergic acid diethylamide. *Science,* **160,** 1343–1344.

Stich, M.S., and Jones, D.S. (1970) Viruses and chromosomes. *Geogr. Med. Virol.,* **12,** 78–127.

Stone, D., Lamson, E., Chang, Y.S., and Pickering, K.W. (1969) Cytogenetic effects of cyclamates on human cells *in vitro. Science,* **164,** 568–569.

Sugimura, T., Nagao, M., Kawachi, T., Honda, M., Yahagi, T., Seino, Y., Sato, S., Matsukura, N., Matsushima, T., Shirai, A., Sawamura, M., and Matsumoto, H. (1977) Mutagen-carcinogens in food, with special reference to highly mutagenic pyrolytic products in broiled foods. In *Origins of Human Cancer* (ed. H.H. Hiatt, J.D. Watson and J.A. Wissten), pp. 1561–1577. (Lab. Cold Spring Harbor).

Suzuki, D.T. (1965) Effects of mitomycin C on crossing-over in *Drosophila melanogaster. Genetics,* **51,** 635–640.

Swietlińska, Z and Zuk, J. (1978) Cytotoxic effects of maleic hydrazide. *Mutat. Res.,* **55,** 15–30.

Tanaka, N., and Sugimura, A. (1956) The effect of azaserine on mitotic cells of *Tradescantia paludosa*, with special reference to restoration and protection against the damage caused by azaserine. *Proc. Int. Genet. Symp.,* 189–195.

Tazima, Y., Kada, T., and Murakami, A. (1975) Mutagenicity of nitrofuran derivatives including furylfuramid, a food preservative. *Mutat. Res.,* **32,** 55–80.

Teas, H.J., and Dyson, J.G. (1967) Mutation in *Drosophila* by methylazoxymethanol, the aglycone of cycasin. *Proc. Soc. Exp. Biol. Med.,* **125,** 988–990.

Teas, H.J., Sax, H.J., and Sax K. (1965) Cycasin: radiomimetic effect. *Science,* **149,** 541–542.

Timson, J. (1977) Caffeine. *Mutat. Res.,* **47,** 1–52.

Tsarapin, L.S. (1966) *Zashch. Vosstanov Luchevykh Povrezhdeniyakh Akad. Nauk SSSR,* **142,** *Chem. Abst.,* **67,** 18400 Y (1967).

Vann, E. (1969) Lethal mutation rate in *Drosophila* exposed to LSD-25 by injection and ingestion. *Nature,* **23,** 95–96.

Vig, B.K. (1971a) Nature of chromosome aberrations induced in pre-DNA synthesis in human leukocytes by daunomycin. *Mutat. Res.,* **12,** 441–452.

Vig, B.K. (1971b) Chromosome aberrations induced in human leukocytes by the antileukemic antibiotic adriamycin. *Cancer. Res.,* **31,** 32–38.

Vig, B.K. (1977) Genetic toxicity of mitomycin C, actionomycin, daunomycin and adriamycin. *Mutat. Res.,* **39,** 189–238.

Vig, B.K., Kontras, S.B., and Samuels, L.D. (1968a) Chromosome aberrations induced by daunomycin in human leukocyte cultures and the apparent synergistic effect of arginine. *Experientia,* **24,** 272–273.

Vig, B.K., Kontras, S.B., Paddock, E.F., and Samuels, L.D. (1968b) Daunomycin-induced chromosomal aberrations and the influence of arginine in modifying the effect of the drug. *Mutat. Res.,* **5,** 279–287.

Vig, B.K., Kontras, S.B., and Aubele, A.M. (1969) Sensitivity of G1 phase of the mitotic cycle to chromosome aberrations induced by daunomycin. *Mutat. Res.,* **7,** 91–97.

Wakonig, R., and Arnason, J.T. (1958) Effects of triazine on chromosomes. *C.R. X Congr. Int. Génét. (Montréal)*, 1958, Vol. II, Abstract 305.

Wassom, J.S., Huff, J.E., and Loprieno, N. (1977–78). A review of the genetic toxicology of chlorinated dibenzo-*p*-dioxins. *Mutat. Res.,* **47,** 141–160.

Wesley, F., Rourke, B., and Darbishire, O. (1965) The formation of persistant toxic chlorhydrins in foodstuffs by fumigation with ethylene oxide and with propylene oxide. *J. Food Sci.,* **30,** 1037–1042.

Wild, D. (1975) Mutagenicity studies on organophosphorus insecticides. *Mutat. Res.,* **32,** 133–150.

Wolff, S., and Luippold, H. (1956) The production of two chemically different types of chromosomal breaks by ionizing radiations. *Proc. Natl. Acad. Sci. USA,* **42,** 510–514.

Wolff, S., Rodin, B., and Cleaver, J.E. (1977) Sister chromaid exchanges induced by mutagenic carcinogens in normal and xeroderma pigmentosum cells. *Nature,* **265,** 347–349.

Zetterberg, G. (1969) Lysergic acid diethylamide and mutation. *Hereditas,* **62,** 262–264.

Zur Hausen, H., and Lanz E. (1966) Chromosomale Aberrationen bei L-Zellen nach Vaccinia-Virus-Infektion. *Z. Med. Mikrobiol. Immunol.,* **152,** 60–65.

Zwelling, L.A., Bradley, M.O., Sharkey, N.A., Anderson, T., and Kohn, K.W. (1979) Mutagenicity, cytotoxicity and DNA crosslinking in V79 Chinese hamster cells treated with *cis-* and *trans-*pt II diamminedichloride. *Mutat. Res.,* **67,** 271–280.

References to Chapter 5

Ames, B.N., Durston, W.E., Yamasaki, E., and Lee, F.D. (1973) Carcinogens are mutagens: a simple test system combining liver homogenates for activation and bacteria for detection. *Proc. Natl. Acad. Sci., USA,* **70**, 2281–2285.

Asquith, J.C., Watts, M.E., Patel, K., Smithen, C.E., and Adams, G.E., (1974) Electron affinic sensitization. V. Radiosensitization of hypoxic bacteria and mammalian cells *in vitro* by some nitroimidazoles and nitropyrazoles. *Radiat. Res.,* **60,** 108–118.

Avanzi, S. (1962) Chromosome breakage in *Vicia faba* by lasiocarpine and monocrotaline. *Caryologia,* **15,** 351–356.

Avers, C.J., and Dryfuss, C.D. (1965) Influence of added nucleosides on acriflavin induction of petite mutants in baker's yeast. *Nature,* **206,** 850.

Bauer, A., Frohberg, H., Jochmann, G., and Schilling, B.U., (1972) Reproduction and mutagenicity trials of 2-methyl-4-nitro-1-(4-nitrophenyl)imidazole. *Naunyn-Schmiedebergs Arch. Pharmacol.,* **274,** R15.

Berget, A., and Weber, T., (1972) Metronidazole and pregnancy. *Ugeskr. Laeg.,* **134,** 2085–2089.

Bick, Y.A.E., and Brown, J.K. (1972) An analysis of chromosomal sensitivity of HPK1 cells from the marsupial *Potorous tridactylus* to X-rays and to heliotrine. *Cytobios,* **5,** 189–200.

Bick, Y.A.E., and Jackson, W.D. (1968) Effects of pyrrolizidine alkaloid heliotrine on cell division and chromosome breakage in cultures of leucocytes from the marsupial *Potorous tridactylus. Aust. J. Biol. Sci.,* **21,** 469.

Bull, L.B. (1955) The histological evidence of liver damage from pyrrolizidine alkaloids. *Aust. Vet. J.,* **31;** 33.

Bull, L.B., Dick, A.T., Keast, J.C., and Edgar, G. (1956) An experimental investigation of the hepatotoxic and other effects on sheep of consumption of *Heliotropium europaeum* L.: heliotrope poisoning in sheep. *Aust. J. Agric. Res.,* **7;** 281.

Buttar, H.S., and Siddiqui, W.H. (1980) Pharmacokinetics and metabolic disposition of ^{14}C-metronidazole-derived radioactivity in rat after intravenous and intravaginal administration. *Arch. Int. Pharmacodyn.,* **245,** 4–19.

Calberg-Bacq, C.M., Delmelle, M., and Duchesne, J. (1968) Inactivation and mutagenesis due to the photodynamic action of acridines and related dyes on extracellular bacteriophage T_4B. *Mutat. Res.,* **6;** 15–24.

Chin, J.B., Sheinin, D.M.K., and Rauth, A.M. (1978) Screening for the mutagenicity of nitro-group containing hypoxic cell radiosensitizers using *Salmonella typhimurium* strains TA 100 and TA 98. *Mutat. Res.*, **58,** 1–10.

Clark, A.M. (1960) The mutagenic activity of some pyrrolizidine alkaloids in *Drosophila. Z. Vererbungsl.*, **91,** 74–80.

Culvenor, C.C.J., Dann, A.T., and Dick, A.T. (1962) Alkylation as the mechanism by which the hepatotoxic pyrrolizidine alkaloids act on cell nuclei. *Nature,* **195,** 570.

D'Amato, F. (1950) Studio statistico dell'attività mutagena dell'acridina e derivati. *Caryologia,* **2,** 229–297.

D'Amato, F. (1951) Nuovi dati sull'attività mutagena dei derivati dell'acridina. *Caryologia,* **3,** 311–326.

D'Amato, F. (1952) Further investigations on the mutagenic activity of acridines. *Caryologia,* **4,** 388–413.

D'Amato, F., and Avanzi, S. (1954) Quarto contributo alla conoscenza dell'attività mutagena dei derivati dell'acridina. *Caryologia,* **6,** 77–89.

De Mars, R.I. (1953) Chemical mutagenesis in bacteriophage T_2. *Nature,* **172,** 964.

Demerec, M., Bertani, G., and Flint, J.A. (1951) A survey of chemicals for mutagenic action on *Escherichia coli. Am. Nat.*, **85,** 119–136.

Dische, S., Saunders, M.I., Lee, M.E., Adams, G.E., and Flockart, I.R. (1977) Chemical testing of the radiosensitizer RO 07-0582. Experience with multiple doses. *Br. J. Cancer,* **35,** 567–576.

Ehrenberg, L., Gustafsson, Å., and Lundqvist, U. (1956) Chemically induced mutation and sterility in barley. *Acta Chem. Scand.*, **10,** 492–494.

Ehrenberg, L., Lundqvist, U., Osterman, S., and Sparrman, B. (1966) On the mutagenic action of alkanesulfonic esters in barley. *Hereditas,* **56,** 277–305.

Feit, P.W. (1960) Synthese der Stereoisomeren 1,2:3,4-dioxido-butane. *Chem. Ber.*, **93,** 116–127.

Feit, P.W. (1961) Stereoisomeren 1,4-di-O-methanesulfonyl-butane-1,2,3,4-tetrole. *Tetrahedron Lett.*, **20,** 716–717.

Feit, P.W. (1964) 1,4-Bismethanesulfonates of the stereoisomeric butane-tetraols and related compounds. *J. Med. Chem.*, **7,** 14–17.

Hartley-Asp, B. (1979) Mutagenicity of metronidazole. *Lancet,* **i,** 275.

Jackson, H., Fox, B.W., and Craig, A.W. (1959) The effect of alkylating agents on male rat fertility. *Br. J. Pharmacol.*, **14,** 149–157.

Kalinowska, E., and Chorazy, M. (1980) Mutagenic activity of some 9-aminoalkyl acridine derivatives on *S. typhimurium. Mutat. Res.*, **78,** 7–15.

Kihlman, B.A. (1959) Induction of structural chromosome changes by visible light. *Nature,* **183,** 976–978.

Korbelik, M., and Horvat, D. (1980) The mutagenicity of nitroaromatic drugs. Effects of metronidazole after incubation in hypoxia *in vitro. Mutat. Res.*, **78,** 201–207.

McCalla, D.R. (1965) Nitrofuran derivatives as radiomimetic agents: cross-resistance studies with *Escherichia coli. Can. J. Microbiol.*, **11,** 185–191.

McCalla, D.R., and Voutsinos, D. (1974) On the mutagenicity of nitrofurans. *Mutat. Res.*, **26,** 3–16.

McKenzie, J.S. (1958) Some pharmacological properties of pyrrolizidine alkaloids and their relationship to chemical structure. *Aust. J. Exp. Biol. Med. Sci.*, **36,** 11.

Moutschen, J. (1965a) Les effets cytogénétiques des composés alkane sulfonates d'alkyl. *Mém. Soc. R. Sci. Liège,* **11,** 113–140.

Moutschen, J. (1965b) Analyse des effets du L-thréitol-1,4,-bis-méthanesulfonate sur les chromosomes de *Vicia faba* L., *Cellule*, **65**, 161–189.

Moutschen, J., and Reekmans, M. (1964) Effects of L-threitol-1,4 bis-methanesulfonate on chromosomes. *Caryologia*, **17**, 495–508. (1964).

Nuti-Ronchi, V., and D'Amato, F. (1961) New data on chromosome breakage by acridine orange in the *Allium* test. *Caryologia,* **14,** 163–165.

Osterman-Golkar, S., Ehrenberg, L., and Wachtmeister, C.A. (1970) Reaction kinetics and biological action in barley of mono-functional methanesulfonic esters. *Radiat. Bot.*, **10**, 303–327.

Ostertag, W., and Kersten, W. (1965) The action of proflavin and actinomycin D in causing chromatid breakage in human cells. *Exp. Cell Res.*, **39**, 296–301.

Schoental, R., and Head, M.A. (1955) Pathological changes in rats as a result of treatment with monocrotaline. *Br. J. Cancer*, **9**, 229.

Schoental, R., and Magee, P.N. (1957) Chronic liver changes in rats after a single dose of lasiocarpine, a pyrrolizidine (*Senecio*), alkaloid. *J. Pathol. Bactiol.*, **74**, 305.

Shahin, M.M. (1982) The dependence of mutagenic activity on chemical structure in two series of related aromatic amines. In *Environmental Mutagens and Carcinogens* (see Sugimura, *et al.* in Gen. Refs.), pp. 379–383.

Shahin, M.M., Bugaut, A., and Kalopissis, G. (1980a) Structure–activity relationship within a series of *m*-diaminobenzene derivatives. *Mutat. Res.*, **78**, 25–31.

Shahin, M.M., Rouers, D., Bugaut, A., and Kalopissis, G. (1980b) Structure–activity relationships within a series of 2,4-diaminoalkyloxybenzene compounds. *Mutat. Res.*, **79**, 289–306.

Shirai, T., and Wang, C.Y. (1980) Enhancement of sister-chromatid exchange in chinese hamster ovary cells by nitrofurans. *Mutat. Res.*, **79**, 345–350.

Speck, W.T., and Rosenkranz, H.S. (1980) Proflavin: an unusual mutagen. *Mutat. Res.*, **77**, 37–43.

Szybalski, W. (1958) Special microbiological systems. II. Observations on chemical mutagenesis in microorganisms. *Ann. N.Y. Acad. Sci.*, **76**, 475–489.

Takanashi, H., Umeda, M., and Hirono, I. (1980) Chromosomal aberrations and mutation in cultured mammalian cells induced by pyrrolizidine alkaloïds. *Mutat. Res.*, **78**, 67–77.

Tazima, Y., Kada, T., and Murakami, A. (1975) Mutagenicity of nitrofuran derivatives, including furylfuramide, a food preservative. *Mutat. Res.*, **32**, 55–80.

Tonomura, A., and Sasaki, M.S. (1973) Chromosome aberration and DNA repair synthesis in cultured human cells exposed to nitrofurans. *Jap. J. Genet.*, **48**, 291–294.

Voogd, C.E., (1981) On mutagenicity of nitroimidazoles. *Mutat. Res.*, **86**, 243–277.

Wardman, P. (1977) The use of nitroaromatic compounds as hypoxic cell radiosensitizers. *Curr. Top. Radiat. Res.*, II, 347–398.

Waterbury, W.E., and Freedman, R. (1964) Induction of phage formation by nitrofurans. *Can. J. Microbiol.*, **10**, 932–934.

Williams, G.M., Mori, H., Hirono, I., and Nagao, M. (1980) Genotoxicity of pyrrolizidine alkaloïds in the hepatocyte primary culture DNA–repair test. *Mutat. Res.*, **79**, 1–5.

Witkin, E.M. (1947) Mutations in *Escherichia coli* induced by chemical agents. *Cold Spring Harbor Symp. Quant. Biol.*, **12**, 256–269.

Woody-Karrer, P., and Greenberg, J. (1963) Resistance and cross-resistance of *Escherichia coli* S mutants to the radiomimetic agent nitrofurazone. *J. Bacteriol.*, **85**, 1208–1216.

Yamanaka, H., Nagao, M., and Sugimura, T. (1979) Mutagenicity of pyrrolizidine alkaloïds in the *Salmonella* mammalian–microsome test. *Mutat. Res.*, **68**, 211–216.

Zampieri, A., and Greenberg, J. (1964) Nitrofurazone as a mutagen in *Escherichia coli*. *Biochem. Biophys. Res. Commun.*, **14**, 172–176.

References to Chapter 6

Abrahamson, S., Bender, M.A., Conger, A.D., and Wolff, S. (1973) Uniformity of radiation – induced mutation rates among different species. *Nature,* **245,** 460–462.

Awa, A.A., and Neriishi, S. (1972) A cytogenetic survey of the offspring of A-bomb survivors in Hiroshima and Nagasaki, Japan. *4th International Conference on Birth Defects, Vienna,* Abstract 92.

Bloom, A.B. (1972) Induced-chromosome aberrations in man. *Adv. Hum. Genet.,* **3,** 99–172.

Brewen, J.G., and Preston, R.J. (1974) Cytogenetic effects of environmental mutagens and the extrapolation to man. *Mutat. Res.,* **26,** 297–305.

Cleaver, J.E. (1968) Defective repair replication of DNA in xeroderma pigmentosum. *Nature,* **218,** 652–656.

Cleaver, J.E. (1977) DNA repair processes and their impairment in some human diseases. In *Progress in Genetic Toxicology* (see Scott *et al.* in Gen. Refs.), pp. 29–39.

Demerec, M., Bertani, G., and Flint, J.A. (1951) A survey of chemicals for mutagenic action on *Escherichia coli. Am. Nat.,* **85,** 119–136.

Ehrenberg, L. (1974) Genetic toxicity of environmental chemicals. *Acta Biol. Iugosl. Ser. F Genetika,* **6,** 367–398.

Evans, H.J. (1977) Molecular mechanisms in the induction of chromosome aberrations. In *Progress in Genetic Toxicology* (see Scott *et al.* in Gen. Refs.) pp. 57–74.

Gilot-Delhalle, J., Thakare, R.G., and Moutschen, J. (1973) Fast rejoining processes in *Nigella damascena* chromosomes revealed by fractionated ^{60}Co γ-ray exposures. *Radiat. Bot.,* **13,** 229–242.

Grahn, D. (1972) Genetic effects of low level irradiation. *Science,* **22,** 535–542.

Green, E.L. (1968) Genetic effects of radiation on mammalian populations. *Annu. Rev. Genet.,* **2,** 87–120.

Holsten, R.D., Sugh, M., and Steward, F.C. (1965) Direct and indirect effects of radiations on plant cells. Their relation to growth and growth induction. *Nature,* **208,** 850–856.

Jensen, K.A., Kirk, I., Kølmark, G., and Westergaard, M. (1951) Chemically induced mutations in *Neurospora. Cold Spring Harbor Symp. Quant. Biol.,* **16,** 245–262.

Kesavan, P.C., and Swaminathan, M.S. (1971) Cytoxic and mutagenic effects of irradiated substrates and food material. *Radiat. Bot.,* **11,** 253–281.

Lea, D.E., and Catcheside, D.G. (1942) The mechanism of the induction by radiation of chromosome aberrations in *Tradescantia. J. Genet.,* **44,** 216–245.

Lejeune, J., Turpin, R., and Rethore, M.O. (1960) Les enfants nés de parents irradiés (cas particuliers de la sex-ratio). *Proc. 9th International Congress Radiology, Munich,* pp. 1089–1096.

Lüning, K.G., and Searle, A.G. (1971) Estimates of the genetic risks from ionizing irradiation. *Mutat. Res.,* **12,** 291–304.

Ma Te-Hsiu, (1968) Effect of irradiated glucose solution on mitotic chromosomes of *Vicia* and *Tradescantia. Radiat. Bot.,* **8,** 307–315.

Moutschen, J. (1968) Some implications of radio-induced structural changes of chromosomes in *Nigella damascena. Nucleus,* **11,** 177–188.

Moutschen, J. (1973) La cytotoxicité et la mutagénicité des aliments irradiés. *Inf. Irradiat. Denrées,* **2,** 51–64.

Moutschen, J., and Matagne, R. (1965) Cytological effects of irradiated glucose. *Radiat. Bot.,* **5,** 23–28.

Moutschen, J., Moutschen-Dahmen, M., and Houbrechts, N. (1976) Cytotoxicité et mutagénicité de deux aldéhydes: crotonaldéhyde et butyraldéhyde chez la souris. *Bull. Soc. R. Sci. Liège,* **45,** 58–72.

Muller, H.J. (1927) Artificial transmutation of the gene. *Science,* **66,** 84–87.

Muller, H.J., (1950) Our load of mutations. *Am. J. Hum. Genet.,* **2,** 111–176.

Muller, H.J. and Altenburg, E. (1919) The rate of change of hereditary factors in *Drosophila. Proc. Soc. Exp. Biol. Med.,* **17,** 10–14.

Neel, J.V., and Schull, W.J. (1956) The effect of exposure to the atomic bombs on pregnancy termination in Hiroshima and Nagasaki. *US Natl. Acad. Sci., Nat. Res. Council,* Publ. 461.

Osterman-Golkar, S., Ehrenberg, L., and Wachtmeister, C.A. (1970) Reaction kinetics and biological action in barley of mono-functional methanesulfonic esters. *Radiat. Bot.,* **10,** 303–327.

Russel, W.L. (1965) Studies in mammalian radiation genetics. *Nucleonics,* **23**, 53–56.

Russel, W.L., Russel, L.B., and Kelly, E.M. (1958) Radiation dose rate and mutation frequency. *Science,* **128,** 1546–1550.

Sasaki, M.S., and Miyata, H. (1968) Biological dosimetry in atomic bomb survivors. *Nature,* **220,** 1189–1193.

Sax, K. (1940) An analysis of X-ray induced chromosome aberrations. *Genetics,* **25,** 41–68.

Sax, K. (1941) Types and frequencies of chromosomal aberrations induced by X-rays. *Cold Spring Harbor Symp. Quant. Biol.,* **9,** 93–103.

Scarascia-Mugnozza, G.T., Natarajan, A.T., and Ehrenberg, L. (1965) *On the Genetic Effects Produced by Irradiated Food Components.* Rapport SEN/IR 15 O.C.D.E., Paris.

Scholte, P.J.L., and Sobels, F.H. (1964) Sex ratio shift among progeny from patients having received therapeutic X-radiation, *Am. J. Hum. Genet.,* **16,** 26–37.

Schöneich, J. (1967) The induction of chromosomal aberrations by hydrogen peroxide in strains of ascites tumors in mice. *Mutat. Res.,* **4,** 385–388.

Schubert, J. (1969) Mutagenicity and cytotoxicity of irradiated food and food components. *Bull. WHO,* **41,** 873–904.

Schull, W.J., and Neel, J.V. (1958) Radiation and the sex-ratio in man. *Science,* **128,** 343–348.

Sedgwick, S.G. (1976) Misrepair of overlapping daughter strand gaps as a possible mechanism for UV induced mutagenesis in UVR strains of *Escherichia coli* a general model for induced mutagenesis by misrepair (SOS repair) of closely spaced DNA lesions. *Mutat. Res.,* **41,** 185–200.

Shaw, M.W., and Hayes, E. (1966) Effects of irradiated sucrose on the chromosomes of human lymphocytes *in vitro. Nature,* **211,** 1254–1256.

Sigler, A.T., Lilienfeld, A.M. Cohen, B.H., and Westlake, J.E. (1965) Radiation exposure in parents with mongolism (Down's syndrome). *Johns Hopkins Med. J.,* **117,** 374.

Smith, R., and von Borstel, R.C. (1972) Genetic control of insect populations. *Science,* **178,** 1164–1174.

Spiher, A.T., Jr. (1968) Food irradiation. *FDA Pap. 2,* No. 8, 15.

Stone, W.S. (1965) Indirect effects of radiation on genetic material. *Brookhaven Symp. Biol.* **8,** 171–190.

Turtóckzy, I., and Ehrenberg, L. (1969) Reaction rates and biological action of alkylating agents. Preliminary report on bactericidal and mutagenic action in *Escherichia coli. Mutat. Res.,* **8,** 229–238.

Vogel, F. (1970) Spontaneous mutation in man. In *Chemical Mutagenesis in Mammals and Man* (see Vogel and Röhrborn in Gen. Refs.), pp. 16–28.

Wagner, R.P., Haddox, C.H., Fuerst, R., and Stone, W.S. (1950) The effect of irradiated medium, cyanide and peroxide on the mutation rate in *Neurospora. Genetics,* **35,** 237–248.

Watson, J., and Schubert, J. (1969) Action of hydrogen peroxide on growth inhibition of *Salmonella typhimurium. Radiat. Res.,* **39,** 554.

Witkin, E. (1976) Ultraviolet mutagenesis and inducible DNA repair in *Escherichia coli. Bacteriol. Rev.,* **40,** 869–907.

Wolff, S., and Luippold, H.E. (1956) The production of two chemically different types of chromosomal breaks by ionizing radiations. *Proc. Natl. Acad. Sci. USA,* **42,** 510–514.

Wyss, O., Stone, W.S., and Clark, J.B. (1947) The production of mutations in *Staphylococcus aureus* by chemical treatment of the substrate. *J. Bacteriol.,* **54,** 767–772.

Wyss, O., Clark, J.B., Haas, F., and Stone, W.S. (1948) The role of peroxide in the biological effects of irradiated broth. *J. Bacteriol.,* **56,** 51–57.

Zelle, M.R., and Hollaender, A. (1955) Effects of radiation on bacteria. In Radiation Biology (see Hollaender in Gen. Refs.), Vol. 2, pp. 365–430.

References to Chapter 7

Adler, I.D., (1980) A review of the coordinated effort on the comparison of test systems for the detection of mutagenic effects, sponsored by the EEC. *Mutat. Res.,* **74,** 77–93.

Ames, B.N. (1976) The detection of carcinogens as mutagens: The Salmonella/ microsome test. In *In Vitro Metabolic Activation in Mutagenesis Testing* (see de Serres, Fouts, Bend, and Philpot in Gen. Refs.), pp. 57–62.

Bateman, A. (1967) A failure to detect any mutagenic action of urethane in the mouse. *Mutat. Res.,* **4,** 710–712.

Bateman, A. (1976) The mutagenic action of urethane. *Mutat. Res.,* **39,** 75–96.

Bridges, B.A. (1975) The mutagenicity of captan and related fungicides. *Mutat. Res.,* **32,** 3–34.

Chollet, M.C., Degraeve, N., Gilot-Delhalle, J., Colizzi, A., Moutschen, J., and Moutschen-Dahmen, M. (1982) Mutagenic efficiency of atrazine with or without mutagenic activation. *Mutat. Res.* **97,** 238 (Abstract).

Dolimpio, D.A., Jacobson, C., and Legator, M. (1968) Effect of aflatoxin on human leukocytes. *Proc. R. Exp. Biol. Med.,* **127,** 559–562.

Eisenbrand, G., Spiegelhalder, B., and Preussmann, R. (1981) Analysis of human biological specimens for nitrosamine contents. In *Banbury Report 7 Gastrointestinal Cancer Endogenous Factors* (eds. W.R. Bruce, P. Correa, M. Lipkin, S.R. Tannenbaum and T.D. Wilkins), pp. 275–283 (Cold Spring Harbor, New York).

Elespuru, R., Setlow, J., and Lijinsky, W. (1973) Nitrosocarbaryl: a new mutagen of environmental significance. *Mutat. Res.,* **21,** 218.

Epstein, S.S., and Shafner, H. (1968) Chemical mutagens in the human environment. *Nature,* **219,** 385–387.

Fahmy, O.G., and Fahmy, M.J. (1968) Mutational mosaicism in relation to dose with the amine and amide derivatives of nitrose compounds in *Drosophila melanogaster. Mutat. Res.,* **6,** 139–154.

Fahmy, O.G., Fahmy, M.J., Massasso, J., and Ondrej, M. (1966) Differential mutagenicity of the amine and amide derivatives of nitroso compounds in *Drosophila melanogaster. Mutat. Res.,* **3,** 201–217.

Fahrig, R. (1971) Metabolic activation of aryldialkyltriazenes in the mouse: induction of mitotic gene conversion in *Saccharomyces cerevisiae* in the host-mediated assay. *Mutat. Res.,* **13,** 436–439.

Fischer, E. (1972) Über die Bildung von Carbaminsaüreäthylester (Urethan) in Getränken nach Behandlung mit Pyrokohlensaürediäthylester. *Lebensm. Untersuch. Forsch.,* **148,** 221–222.

Freese, E., Sklarow, S., and Freese, E.B. (1968) DNA damage caused by antidepressant hydrazines and related drugs. *Mutat. Res.,* **5,** 343–347.

Gabridge, H.G., and Legator, M.S. (1969) A host-mediated microbial assay for the detection of mutagenic compounds. *Proc. Soc. Exp. Biol. Med.,* **130**, 831–839.

Geissler, E. (1962) Über die Wirkung von Nitrosaminen auf Mikroorganismen. *Naturwissenschaften,* **49,** 380–381.

Gentile, J.M., and Plewa, M.J. (1981) The maize-microbe bioassay. A unique approach to environmental mutagenesis. In *In Vitro Toxicity Testing of Environmental Agents,* Proceedings NATO Advanced Research Institute, Monte Carlo.

Green, S., Legator, M.S., and Jacobson, C. (1967) Utilization of a cell line derived from rat kangaroo for cytogenetic studies. *Mammalian chromosomes Newsletter*, **8,** 36.

Hartman, P.E. (1982) Nitrates and nitrites: Ingestion, pharmacodynamics, toxicology. In *Chemical Mutagens* (see de Serres and Hollaender in Gen. Refs.), Vol. 7, pp. 211–294.

Hill, M.J., Hawksworth, G., and Tattersall, G. (1973) Bacteria, nitrosamines and cancer of the stomach. *Br. J. Cancer,* **28,** 562–567.

Hussain, S., and Ehrenberg, L. (1974) Mutagenicity of primary amines combined with nitrite. *Mutat. Res.,* **26,** 419–422.

Kada, T., Morita, K., and Inone, T. (1978) Antimutagenic action of vegetable factors on the mutagenic principle of tryptophane pyrolysate. *Mutat. Res.,* **53,** 351–353.

Legator, M.S. (1966) Biological effects of aflatoxin in cell culture. *Bacteriol. Rev.,* **30,** 471–477.

Legator, M.S., and Verrett, J. (1967) Conference on Biological Effects of Pesticides in Mammalian Systems. Abstract No. 6, p. 17. N.Y. Acad. Sci.

Lijinsky, W. (1974) Reaction of drugs with nitrous acid as a source of carcinogenic nitrosamines. *Cancer Res.,* **34,** 255–258.

Lijinsky, W., Loo, J., and Ross, A.E. (1968) Mechanism of alkylating of nucleic acids by nitrosodimethylamine. *Nature (London),* **218,** 1174–1175.

Lilly, L.J. (1965) Induction of chromosome aberrations by aflatoxin. *Nature,* **207,** 433–434.

Löfroth, G., and Gejvall, T. (1971) Diethyl pyrocarbonate: formation of urethan in treated beverages. *Science,* **174,** 1248–1250.

Lukens, R.J., and Sisler, H.D. (1958) Chemical reactions involved in the fungitoxicity of captan. *Phytopathology,* **48,** 235.

Malling, H.V. (1966) Mutagenicity of two potent carcinogens, dimethylnitrosamine and diethylnitrosamine in *Neurospora crassa. Mutat. Res.,* **3,** 537–540.

Malling, H.V. (1971) Dimethylnitrosamine. Formation of mutagenic compounds by interaction with mouse liver microsomes. *Mutat. Res.,* **13,** 425–429.

Marquardt, H., Zimmermann, F.K., and Schwaier, R. (1964) Die Wirkung krebsauslösender Nitrosamine und Nitrosamide auf das Adenin-6-45-Rückmutationssystem von *Saccharomyces cerevisiae. Z. Vererbungsl.,* **95,** 82–96.

Morita, K., Hara, M., and Kada, T. (1978) Studies on natural desmutagens: Screening for vegetable and fruit factors active in inactivation of mutagenic pyrolysis products from animal acids. *Agric. Biol. Chem.,* **42,** 1235–1238.

Moulé, Y., Moreau, S., and Bousquet, J.F. (1977) Relationships between the chemical structure and the biological properties of some eremophilane compounds related to PR toxin. *Chem. Biol. Interact.,* **17,** 185–192.

Moulé, Y., Moreau, S., and Aujaer, C. (1980) Induction of cross-links between DNA and protein by PR toxin, a mycotoxin from *Penicillium roqueforti. Mutat. Res.,* **77,** 79–89.

Moulé, Y., Decloitre, F., and Hamon, G. (1981a) Mutagenicity of the mycotoxin Botryodiplodin in the *Salmonella typhimurium*/microsomal activation test. *Environ. Mutagenesis,* **3,** 287–291.

Moulé, Y., Douce, C., Moreau, S., and Darracq, N. (1981b) Effects of the mycotoxin botryodiplodin on mammalian cells in culture. *Chem. Biol. Interact.,* **37,** 155–164.

Oehlkers, F. (1943) Die Auslösung von Chromosomenmutation in der Meiosis durch die Einwirkung von Chemikalien. *Z. Indukt. Abstamm. Vererbungsl.,* **81,** 313–341.

Oehlkers, F. (1953) Chromosome breaks influenced by chemicals. Symposium on chromosome breakage. *Heredity*, **6,** (*Suppl.*;, 95–105.

Ong, T. (1970) Mutagenicity of aflatoxin in *Neurospora crassa. Mutat. Res.,* **9,** 615–618.

Ong, T. (1975) Aflatoxin mutagenesis. *Mutat. Res.*, **32**, 35–53.

Ong, T., and de Serres, F.J. (1971) Mutagenicity of 1-phenyl-3,3-dimethyltriazene and 1-phenyl-3-monomethyltriazene in *Neurospora crassa. Mutat. Res.*, **13**, 276–278.

Owens, R.G., and Novotny, H.M. (1959) Mechanism of action of the fungicide: captan (*N*-(trichloromethylthio)-4-cyclohexene-1,2-dicarboximide). *Contrib. Boyce Thompson Inst.*, **20**, 171–190.

Pasternak, L. (1962) Mutagen Wirkung von Dymethylnitrosamin bei *Drosophila melanogaster. Naturwissenschaften,* **49**, 381.

Pasternak, L. (1963) Untersuchangen über die mutagene Wirkung von Nitrosamin und Nitrosomethyl-harnstoff. *Acta Biol. Med. Ger.*, **10**, 436.

Pasternak, L. (1964) Untersuchungen über die mutagen Wirkung verschiedener Nitrosamin- und nitrosamid-Verbindungen. *Arzneim. Forsch.*, **14**, 802–804.

Plewa, M.J., and Gentile, J.M. (1975) A maize-microbe bioassay for the detection of proximal mutagenicity of agricultural chemicals. *Maize Genet. Coop. Newslett.*, **49**, 40–43.

Plewa, M.J., and Gentile, J.M. (1976a) Plant activation of herbicides into environmental mutagens. The *waxy* reversion bioassay. *Maize Genet. Coop. Newslett.* **50**, 44.

Plewa, M.J., and Gentile, J.M. (1976b) Mutagenicity of atrazine. A maize-microbe bioassay. *Mutat. Res.*, **38**, 287–292.

Plewa, M.J., and Gentile, J.M. (1982) The activation of chemicals into mutagens by green plants. In *Chemical Mutagens* (see de Serres and Hollaender in Gen. Refs.) Vol. 7, pp. 401–420.

Pogodina, O.N. (1966) O mutagennoy aktivnosti Kancerogenov iz gruppy nitrosaminov. *Citologya,* **8**, 503–509.

Preussmann, R. (1968, 1969) Zum Wirkungmechanismus karzinogener Aryldialkyltriazene. Fortschritte der Krebsforschung. In *Bericht über die 10 Wissenschaftliche Tagung des Deutschen Zentralausschusses für Krebsbekämpfung und Krebsforschung* (Berlin), pp. 163–169.

Preussmann, R., von Hodenberg, A., and Hengy, H. (1969) Mechanism of carcinogenesis with 1-aryl-3,3-dialkyl-triazenes. Enzymatic dealkylation by rat liver microsomal fraction *in vitro. Biochem. Pharmacol.*, **18**, 1–13.

Radomski, J.L., Greenwald, D., Hearn, W.L., Block, N.L. and Woods, F.M. (1978) Nitrosamine formation in bladder infections and its role in the etiology of bladder cancer. *J. Urol.*, **120**, 48–50.

Rapoport, I.A. (1948) Acylation of genic molecules. *Dokl. Akad. Nauk SSSR,* **55**, 1183–1186 (in Russian).

Rapaport, I.A. (1948) Supermutagens (in Russian with English summaries). Nauk (Moscow).

Roberts, G.T., and Allen, J.W. (1980) Tissue-specific induction of sister chromatid exchanges by ethyl carbamate. *Environ. Mutagenesis,* **2**, 17–26.

Röhrborn, G., Proping, P., and Buselmaier, W. (1972) Mutagenic activity of isoniazid and hydrazide in mammalian test systems. *Mutat. Res.*, **16**, 189–194.

Russel, W., Kelly, E.M., Hunsicker, P.R., Bangham, J.W., Maddux, S.C., and Phipps, E.L. (1979) Specific-locus test shows ethylnitrosourea to be the most potent mutagen in the mouse. *Proc. Natl. Acad. Sci. USA,* **76**, 5818–5819.

Scott, B.R., Sparrow, A.H., Schwemmer, J.S., and Schairer, A. (1978) Plant metabolic activation of 1,2-dibromomethane (EDB) to a mutagen of greater potency. *Mutat. Res.*, **49**, 203–212.

Veleminsky, J., and Gichner, T. (1968) The mutagenic activity of nitrosamines in *Arabidopsis thaliana. Mutat. Res.*, **5**, 429–431.

Vogel, E. (1971) Chemische Konstitution und mutagene Wirkung. VI. Induktion dominanter und rezessiv-geschlechtsgebundener Letalmutationen durch Aryldialkyltriazene bei *Drosophila melanogaster. Mutat. Res.*, **11**, 397–410.

Vogel, E., Fahrig, R., and Obe, G. (1973) Triazenes: a new group of indirect mutagens.

Comparative investigations of the genetic effects of different aryldiakyltriazenes using *Saccharomyces cerevisiae,* the host-mediated assay, *Drosophila melanogaster* and human chromosomes *in vitro. Mutat. Res.,* **21,** 123–136.

Wei, R.D., Still, P.E., Smalley, E.B., Schnoes, H.K., and Strong, F.M. (1973) Isolation and partial characterization of a mycotoxin from *Penicillium roqueforti. Appl. Microbiol.,* **25,** 111.

Wei, R.D., Schnoes, H.K., Hart, P.A., and Strong, F.M. (1975) The structure of PR toxin in a mycotoxin from *Penicillium roqueforti. Tetrahedron,* **31,** 109.

Wei, R.D., Ong, T.M, Whong, W.Z., Frezza, D., Bronzetti, G., and Zeiger, E., (1979) Genetic effects of PR toxin in eukaryotic micro-organism. *Environ. Mutagenesis,* **1,** 45–53.

Yano, K. (1979) Effect of vegetable juices and milk on alkylating activity of *N*-methyl-*N*-nitrosourea. *Agric. Food Chem.,* **27,** 456–458.

References to Chapter 8

Åberg, B., Ekman, L., and Falk, R. (1969) Metabolism of methyl mercury (^{203}Hg) compounds in man. *Arch. Environ. Health,* **19,** 478–484.

Bari, G. (1963) The mutagenic effect of ethyl methane sulfonate alone and in combination with copper on wheat. *Caryologia,* **16,** 619–624.

Bhatia, C.R., and Narayanan, K.R. (1965) Genetic effects of ethyl methane sulfonate in combination with copper and zinc ion on *Arabidopsis thaliana. Genetics,* **52,** 577–581.

Brøgger, A. (1974) Caffeine-induced enhancement of chromosome damage in human lymphocytes treated with methyl methane sulphonate mitomycin and X-rays. *Mutat. Res.,* **23,** 353–360.

Chrisp, C.E., and Fisher, G.L. (1980) Mutagenicity of airborne particles. *Mutat. Res.,* **76,** 143–164.

Conney, A.H. (1967) Pharmacological implications of microsomal enzyme induction. *Pharmacol. Rev.,* **19,** 317.

Degraeve, N. (1967) Influence du bichlorure de mercure sur les effets du méthane sulfonate d'éthyl au niveau chromosomique. *Bull. Soc. R. Bot. Belg.,* **100,** 41–50.

Degraeve, N. (1981) Carcinogenic, teratogenic and mutagenic effects of cadmium. *Mutat. Res.,* **86,** 115–135.

Demarini, D.M. (1978) The mutagenicity of cigarette smoke condensate in *Saccharomyces cerevisiae. Mutat. Res.,* 53–84.

Demarini, D.M. (1979) The mutagenicity of cigarette smoke condensate in *Neurospora crassa. 10th Annu. Meeting Environ. Mutagen.* p. 40 (Abstract)

De Raat, W.K. (1979) Comparison of the induction by cigarette condensates of sister chromatid exchanges in Chinese hamster ovary cells and of mutations in *Salmonella typhimurium. Mutat. Res.,* **66,** 253–259.

Fahmy, F.Y. (1951) Cytogenetic analysis of the action of some fungicide mercurials. *Ph.D. Thesis.* Institute of Genetics, University of Lund (Sweden).

Fiskesjö, G. (1969) Some results from *Allium* tests with organic mercury halogenides. *Hereditas,* **62,** 314–322.

Fiskesjö, G. (1970) The effect of two organic mercury compounds on human leukocytes *in vitro. Hereditas,* **64,** 142–146.

Gasiorek, K., and Bauchinger, M. (1981) Chromosome changes in lymphocytes after separate and combined treatments with divalent salts of lead, cadmium and zinc. *Environ. Mutagenesis,* **3,** 513–518.

Gerber, G.B., Léonard, A., and Jacquet, P. (1980) Toxicity, mutagenicity and teratogenicity of lead. *Mutat. Res.,* **76,** 115–141.

Ghazal, A., Koransky, W., Portig, J., Vohland, H.W., and Klempaw, I. (1964) Beschleunigung von Entgiftungsreaktionen durch verschiedene Insecticiden. *Arch. Exp. Pathol. Pharmakol.,* **249,** 1–10.

Gilot, J., Moutschen, J., and Moutschen-Dahmen, M. (1967) Mutagenesis with ethyl methanesulphonate in *Nigella damascena* L. *Experientia,* **23,** 673.

Hartman, P. (1983) Putative mutagens and carcinogens in foods. Sorbate and sorbate-nitrite interactions. *Environ. Mutagenesis,* **5,** 217–222.

Henderson, T.R., Li, A.P., Royer, R.E., and Clark, C.R. (1981) Increased cytotoxicity and mutagenicity of diesel fuel after reaction with NO_2. *Environ. Mutagenesis,* **3,** 211–220.

Hixon, S.C., and Yielding, N.L. (1976) A protective effect of caffeine on the ethidium induced petite mutation in yeast. *Mutat. Res.,* **34,** 195–200.

Hughes, T.J., Pellizzari, Little, L., Sparacino, C., and Kolber, A. (1980) Ambient air pollutants: collection, chemical, characterization and mutagenicity testing. *Mutat. Res.,* **76,** 51–83.

Jensen, S., and Jernelöv, A. (1969) Biosynthesis of mono- and dimethyl-mercury. *Nature,* **223,** 1453–1454.

Kada, T. (1973) DNA-damaging products from reaction between sodium nitrite and sorbic acid. *Annu. Rept. Natl. Inst. Genet.,* **24,** 43.

King, K.C., Kohan, M.J., Austin, A.C., Claxton, L.D., and Huisingh, J.L. (1981) Evaluation of the release of mutagens from diesel particles in the presence of physiological fluids. *Environ. Mutagenesis,* **3,** 109–121.

Kostoff, D. (1939) Effect of the fungicide 'Granosan' on atypical growth and chromosome doubling in plants. *Nature,* **144,** 334.

Kostoff, D. (1940) Atypical growth, abnormal mitosis and polyploidy induced by ethylmercurychloride. *Phytopathol. Z.,* **23,** 90–96.

Kuhlmann, W., Fromme, H.G., Heege, E.M., and Ostertag, W. (1968) The mutagenic action of caffeine in higher organisms. *Cancer Res.,* **28,** 2375–2389.

Léonard, A., and Lauwerys, R.R. (1980a) Carcinogenicity, teratogenicity and mutagenicity of arsenic. *Mutat. Res.* **75,** 49–62.

Léonard, A., and Lauwerys, R.R. (1980b) Carcinogenicity and mutagenicity of chromium. *Mutat. Res.,* **76,** 227–239.

Léonard, A., Gerber, G.B., and Jacquet, P. (1981) Carcinogenicity, mutagenicity and teratogenicity of nickel. *Mutat. Res.,* **87,** 1–15.

Léonard, A., Jacquet, P., and Lauwerys, R.R. (1983) Mutagenicity and teratogenicity of mercury compounds. *Mutat. Res.,* **114,** 1–18.

Lieb, M. (1961) Enhancement of ultraviolet-induced mutation in bacteria by caffeine. *Z Vererbungsl.,* **92,** 416–429.

Loper, J. (1980) Mutagenic effects of organic compounds in drinking water. *Mutat. Res.,* **76**, 241–268.

Lower, W., Rose, P., and Drobney, V. (1978) *In situ* mutagenic and other effects associated with lead smelting. *Mutat. Res.,* **54**, 83–93.

MacFarlane, E.W.E. (1950) Somatic mutations produced by organic mercurials in flowering plants. *Genetics,* **35,** 122–123.

McLean, A.E.M. (1965) Pesticides and food additives. *Lancet,* **18**, 1295.

Moriyama, H. (1968) A study on congenital Minamata disease. *Kumamoto Igakkai Zasshi,* **41,** 506–532.

Moutschen, J. (1965) Les effets cytogénétiques des composés alkane sulfonates d'alkyl. *Mem. Soc. R. Sci. Liège,* **11**, 1–296.

Moutschen, J., and Moutschen-Dahmen, M. (1963a) Influence of Cu^{++} and Zn^{++} ions on the effects of ethyl methanesulfonate (EMS) on chromosomes. *Experientia,* **19,** 144–147.

Moutschen, J., and Moutschen-Dahmen, M. (1963b) Interactions ioniques dans les effets radiomimétiques du méthane sulfonate d'éthyl (EMS) sur les chromosomes de *Vicia faba. Radiat. Bot.,* **3,** 297–310.

Moutschen, J., Moutschen-Dahmen, M., and Degraeve, N. (1965) Modified effects of ethyl methane sulfonate (EMS) at the chromosome level. In *Mechanism of Mutation and Inducing Factors,* (ed. A. Lengerová), *Proc. Symp. Mutational Process* (Prague), pp. 397–400.

Nemirovskii, L.E., and Klimenko, V.V. (1973) Effect of caffeine on genetic lesions induced by the alkylating compound dipine on hepatocytes of rats. *Genetika,* **9,** 100–106.

Norén, K., and Westöo, G. (1967) Methyl mercury in fish. *Vår Föda,* **19,** 13–17.

Pescitelli, A.R. (1979) Mutagenicity of cigarette smoke condensate and cigarette smoke in *Drosophila melanogaster. 10th Annu. Meet. Environ. Mutagen,* p. 40.

Plewa, M., and Gentile, J. (1976) Mutagenicity of atrazine: A maize:microbe bioassay. *Mutat. Res.,* **38,** 287–292.

Ramel, C. (1969) Genetic effects of organic mercury compounds. I. Cytological investigations on *Allium* roots. *Hereditas,* **61,** 208–230.

Ramel, C., and Magnusson, J. (1969) Genetic effects of organic mercury compounds. II. Chromosome segregation in *Drosophila melanogaster. Hereditas,* **61,** 231–254.

Rauth, A.M. (1967) Evidence for dark-reaction of ultraviolet light damage in mouse L-cells. *Radiat. Res.,* **31,** 121–138.

Schairer, L., Van't Hof, J., Hayes, C., Burton, R., and de Serres, F.J. (1978a) Measurement of biological activity of ambient air mixtures using a mobile laboratory for *in situ* exposures — preliminary results from the *Tradescantia* plant test system. In *Application of Short-term Bioassays in the Fractionation and Analysis of Complex Environmental Mixtures,* EPA Publ. 600/9-78-027, pp. 419–440.

Schairer, L., Van't Hof, J., Hayes, C., Burton, R., and de Serres, F.J. (1978b) Exploratory monitoring of air pollutants for mutagenic activity with the *Tradescantia* stamen hair system. *Environ. Health Perspect.,* **27,** 51–60.

Skerfving, S., Hansson, K. and Lindsten, J. (1970) Chromosome breakage in humans exposed to methyl mercury through fish consumption. *Arch. Environ. Health,* **21,** 133–139.

Tazima, Y. (1982) A brief sketch of environmental mutagen studies in Japan. In *Environmental Mutagens and Carcinogens* (see Sugimura *et al.* in Gen. Refs.), pp. 91–100.

Timson, J. (1977) Caffeine. *Mutat. Res.,* **47,** 1–52.

Van't Hof, J., and Schairer, L.A. (1982) *Tradescantia* assay system for gaseous mutagens. A Report of the U.S. Environmental Protection Agency Gene-Tox Program. *Mutat. Res.,* **99,** 303–315.

Wakabayashi, K., Yahagi, T., Nagao, M., and Sugimura, T. (1982) Comutagenic effect of norharman with aminopyrine derivatives. *Mutat. Res.,* **105,** 205–210.

Westöo, G. (1967) Mercury in fish. *Vår Föda,* **19,** 1–7.

Whong, W.Z., Stewart, J., McCawley, M., Major, P., Merchant, J.A., and Ong, T. (1981) Mutagenicity of airborne particles from a nonindustrial town. *Environ. Mutagenesis,* **3,** 617–626.

Witkin, E.M. (1958) Post-irradiation metabolism and the timing of ultraviolet-induced mutations in bacteria. *C.R. Xe Congr. Int. Génét. (Montreal),* **1,** 280–299.

World Health Organization (1963) Air pollution, 1–456 (Geneva).

Wragg, J.B., Carr, J.V., and Ross, V. (1967) Inhibition of DNA polymerase activity by caffeine in a mammalian cell line. *J. Cell Biol.,* **35,** 146A–147A.

Zavon, M.R. (1969) Interactions. *Bioscience,* **19,** 892–895.

References to Chapter 9

Ames, B.N., McCann, J., and Yamasaki, E. (1977) Methods for detecting carcinogens and mutagens with the *Salmonella*/mammalian–microsome test. In Handbook of

Mutagenicity Test Procedures (see Kilbey, Legator and Ramel in Gen. Refs.), pp. 1–17.

Beatty, R.A. (1977) F-bodies as Y chromosome markers in nature human sperm heads. A quantitative approach. *Cytogenet. Cell. Genet.*, **18,** 33–49.

Browning, L.S. (1973) Mutagenicity of various chemicals and their metabolites in *Drosophila. Genetics,* **74,** 533.

Chebotarer, A.N., Telegin, L.Y., and Derzharets, E.M. (1976) Cytogenetic effect of cyclophosphamide in human lymphocyte culture after its activation in mice. *Genetika,* **10,** 151–157.

Clayson, D.B. (1980) ICPEMC working paper 2/1. Comparison between *in vitro* and *in vivo* tests for carcinogenicity. An overview. *Mutat. Res.,* **75,** 205–213.

Connor, T.H., Cantelli-Forti, G., Sitra, P., and Legator, M.S. (1979) Bile as a source of mutagenic metabolites produced *in vivo* and detected by *Salmonella typhimurium. Environ. Mutagenesis,* **1,** 269–276.

David, G., Bisson, J.P., Czysik, F., Jouannet, P., and Gernigon, G. (1975) Anomalies morphologiques du spermatozoïde humain. *J. Gynécol. Obstét. Biol. Reprod.,* **4,** (*Suppl.*) 17–36.

Durston, W.E., and Ames, B.N. (1974) A simple method for the detection of mutagens in urine. Studies with carcinogen 2-acetyl-aminofluorene. *Proc. Natl. Acad. Sci. USA.,* **71,** 737–741.

Ehrenberg, L. (1973) The relation of cancer induction and genetic damage. In *Evaluation of Genetic Risks of Environmental Chemicals, Ambio Special Report,* (ed. C. Ramel), Vol. 3, pp. 15–16. (Stockholm).

Ehrenberg, L., and Osterman-Golkar, S. (1980) Alkylation of macromolecules for detecting mutagenic agents. *Teratogenesis, Carcinogenesis Mutagenesis,* **1,** 105–127.

Ehrenberg, L., Hiesche, K.D., Osterman-Golkar, S., and Wennberg, I. (1974) Evaluation of genetic risks of alkylating agents: Tissue doses in the mouse from air contaminated with ethylene oxide. *Mutat. Res.*, **24,** 83–103.

Foster, R.E., and Rostenbach, R.E. (1954) Distribution of radioisotopes in the Columbia river. *J. Am. Water Works Assoc.,* **46,** 640–663.

Grant, W.F. (1970) Pesticides and heredity. *MacDonald, J.,* **31,** 211–214.

Grant, W.F. (1972) Pesticides — Subtle promoters of evolution. *Symp. Biol. Hung.,* **12,** 43–50.

Gustafsson, Å. (1972) Poisoning the earth. *Nord. Försäkrings Tidsk.,* **3,** 231–236.

Kapp, R.W., and Jacobson, C.B. (1980) Analysis of human spermatozoa for Y chromosomal non disjunction. *Teratogenesis, Carcinogenesis, Mutagenesis*, **1,** 193–211.

Kilian, D.J., and Picciano, D. (1976) Cytogenetic surveillance of industrial populations. In *Chemical Mutagens* (see Hollaender in Gen. Refs.), Vol. 4, pp. 321–339.

Kostoff, D. (1931) Heteroploidy in *Nicotiana tabacum* and *Solanum melongena* caused by fumigation with nicotine sulphate. *Bull. Soc. Bot. Bulg.,* **4,** 87–92.

Kuhnlein, U., Bergström, D., and Kuhnlein, H. (1981) Mutagens in feces from vegetarians and non vegetarians. *Mutat. Res.,* **85,** 1–12.

Legator, J.S., Truong, L., and Connor, T.H. (1978) Analysis of body fluids including alkylation of macromolecules for detection of mutagenic agents. In *Chemical Mutagens* (see Hollaender and de Serres in Gen. Refs.), Vol. 5, pp. 1–23.

Mann, J.D., and Storey, W.B. (1966) Rapid action of carbamate herbicides upon plant cell nuclei. *Cytologia,* **31,** 203–207.

Markarian, D.S. (1967) Effects of dieldrin on the mitosis in *Crepis capillaris* sprouts. *Genetika,* **1,** 132–137.

Mellanby, K. (1972) Effects of pollution on wild life in Britain. In *Population and Pollution* (eds. (P.R. Cox and S. Peel), pp. 45–51. Academic Press (London and New York).

Oesch, F., Bentley, P., And Glatt, H. (1976) Prevention of benzo(*a*)pyrene-induced mutagenicity by homogenous epoxide hydratase. *Int. J. Cancer,* **18,** 448–452.

Oesch, F., Raphael, D., Schwind, H., and Glatt, H.R. (1977) Species differences in activating and inactivating enzymes related to the control of mutagenic metabolites. *Arch. Toxicol.,* **39,** 97–108.

Osterman-Golkar, S., Ehrenberg, L., Segerbäck, D., and Hällström, I. (1976) Evaluation of genetic risks of alkylating agents. II. Haemoglobin as a dose monitor. *Mutat. Res.,* **34,** 1–10.

Osterman-Golkar, S., Hultmark, D., Segerbäck, D., Calleman, C.J., Göthe, R., Ehrenberg, L., and Wachtmeister, C.A. (1977) Alkylation of DNA and proteins in mice exposed to vinyl chloride. *Biochem. Biophys. Res. Commun.,* **76,** 259–266.

Rannug, U., and Beije, B. (1978) The mutagenic effect of 1,2-dichloroethane on *Salmonella typhimurium.* II. Activation by the isolated perfused rat liver. *Chem. Biol. Interact.,* **24,** 265–285.

Scheline, R.R. (1973) Metabolism of foreign compounds by gastrointestinal microorganisms. *Pharmacol. Rev.,* **25,** 441–532.

Schmähl, D., and Pool, B.L. (1982) What is the predictive value of short-term mutagenicity testing to determine carcinogenic potential of compounds? In *Environmental Mutagens and Carcinogens* (see Sugimura *et al.* in Gen. Refs.), pp. 295–303.

Segerbäck, D., Calleman, C.J., Ehrenberg, L., Löfroth, G., and Osterman-Golkar, S. (1978) Evaluation of genetic risks of alkylating agents. IV. Quantitative determination of alkylated amino acids in haemoglobin as a measure of the dose after treatment of mice with methyl methanesulfonate. *Mutat. Res.,* **49,** 71–82.

Siebert, D. (1973) A new method for testing genetically active metabolites. Urinary assay wih cyclophosphamide (Endoxan, Cytoxan) and *Saccharomyces cerevisiae. Mutat. Res.,* **17,** 307–314.

Siebert, D., and Simon, U. (1973a) Cyclophosphamide: pilot study of genetically active metabolites in the urine of a treated human patient. Induction of mitotic gene conversions in yeast. *Mutat. Res.,* **19,** 65–72.

Siebert, D., and Simon, U. (1973b) Genetic activity of metabolites in the ascitic fluid and on the urine of human patient treated with cyclophosphamide: Induction of mitotic gene conversion in *Saccharomyces cerevisiae. Mutat. Res.,* **21,** 257–262.

Stebbins, G.L. (1959) Genes, chromosomes and evolution. In *Vistas in Botany* (ed. W.B. Turril), pp. 258–290. Pergamon Press (New York).

Strong, L.C. (1948) The induction of mutations by a carcinogen. Proc. VIIth Intl. Congr. Genet. *Hereditas,* (*Suppl.*), 486–499.

Van Den Born, W.H. (1969) Picloram residues and crop production. *Can. J. Plant Sci.,* **49,** 628–629.

Weisburger, J.H., and Williams, G.M. (1982) Classification of carcinogens as genotoxic and epigenetic as basis for improved toxicologic bioassay methods. In *Environmental Mutagens and Carcinogens* (see Sugimura *et al.* in Gen. Refs.), pp. 283–294.

Wright, A.S. (1980) ICPM working paper 2/2. The role of metabolism in chemical mutagenesis and chemical carcinogenesis. *Mutat. Res.,* **75,** 215–241.

References to Chapter 10

Alekperov, U. (1982) Antimutagens and the problem of controlling the action of environmental mutagens. In *Environmental Mutagens and Carcinogens* (see Sugimura *et al.* in Gen. Refs.), pp. 361–368.

Batzinger, R., Bueding, E., Crawford, K., and Bruce, J. (1979) Prevention of the mutagenic activation of an antischistosomal isothiocyanate in primates by an antibiotic. *Environ. Mutagenesis,* **1,** 353–360.

Bochkov, N.B., Sram, R.J., Kuleshov, N.P., and Zhurkov, V.S. (1976) System for the evaluation of the risk from chemical mutagens for man. Basic principles and practical recommendations. *Mutat. Res.,* **38,** 191–202.

Bridges, B.A. (1973) Some general principles of mutagenicity screening and a possible framework for testing procedures. *Environ. Health Perspect.,* **6,** 221–227.

Dean, B.J. (1976) A predictive testing scheme for carcinogenicity and mutagenicity of industrial chemicals. *Mutat. Res.,* **41,** 83–88.

Degraeve, N. (1967) Influence du bichlorure de mercure sur les effets du méthane sulfonate d'éthyl au niveau chromosomique. *Bull. Soc. Ry. Bot. Belg.,* **100,** 41–50.

Ehrenberg, L., Gustafsson, Å., and Lundqvist, U. (1956) Chemically induced mutation and sterility in barley. *Acta Chem. Scand.,* **10,** 492–494.

Ehrenberg, L., Hiesche, K.D., Osterman-Golkar, S., and Wennberg, I. (1974) Evaluation of genetic risks of alkylating agents: tissue doses in the mouse from air contaminated with ethylene oxide. *Mutat. Res.,* **24,** 83–103.

Haynes, R.H. and Eckardt, F. (1980) Mathematical analysis of mutation-induction kinetics. In *Chemical Mutagens.* (see de Serres and Hollaender in Gen. Refs.), Vol. 6, pp. 271–307.

Hollstein, M., McCann J., Angelosanto, F.A., and Nichols, W.W. (1979) Short term tests for carcinogens and mutagens. *Mutat. Res.,* **65,** 133–226.

Jansen, J.D., Clemmesen, J., and Sundaram, K. (1980) Isoniazid: An attempt at retrospective prediction. ICPEMC Publication No. 4. *Mutat. Res.,* **76,** 85–112.

Johnson, H.G., and Bach, M.K. (1965) Apparent suppression of mutation rates in bacteria by spermine. *Nature,* **208,** 408–409.

Kada, T. (1982) Mechanisms and genetic implications of environmental antimutagens. In *Environmental Mutagens and Carcinogens* (see Sugimura, *et al.* in Gen. Refs.), pp. 357–359.

Kada, T., Morita, K., and Inoue, T. (1978) Anti-mutagenic action of vegetable factor(s) on the mutagenic principle of tryptophan pyrolysate. *Mutat. Res.,* **53,** 351–353.

Kaplan, W.D., and Lyon, M.F. (1953a) Failure of mercaptoethylamine to protect against the mutagenic effects of radiation. I. Experiments with *Drosophila. Science,* **118,** 776–777.

Kaplan, W.D., and Lyon, M.F. (1953b) Failure of mercaptoethylamine to protect against the mutagenic effects of radiation. II. Experiments with mice. *Science,* **118,** 777–778.

Kimball, R.F. (1977) The mutagenicity of hydrazine and some of its derivatives. *Mutat. Res.,* **39,** 111–126.

Komura, H., Minakata, H., Nakanishi K., Mochizuki, H., and Kada, T. (1981) Chemical features of antimutagenic factor in human placenta. *3rd Int. Conf. Env. Mutagens* (Tokyo) 3B18 (Abstract) 83.

Legator, M., and Zimmering, S. (1975) Integration of mammalian, microbial and *Drosophila* procedures for evaluating chemical mutagens. *Mutat. Res.,* **29,** 181–188.

Mikaelsen, K. (1952) The protective effect of glutathione against radiation induced chromosome aberrations. *Science,* **116,** 172–174.

Moës, A. (1957) L'action de la cystéamine chez l'orge. *Bull. Inst. Agron. Stn. Rech. Gembloux,* **25,** 98–107.

Molineaux, C.J., Batzinger, R.P., Schmidt, W., and Baeding, E. (1980) Mutagenic activation of an antischistosomal drug by enteric *Streptococcus* sps *in vitro* and *in vivo*. *Teratogenesis, Carcinogenesis, Mutagenesis,* **1,** 129–139.

Morita, K., Hara, M., and Kada, T. (1978) Studies on natural desmutagens: Screening for vegetable and fruit factors active in inactivation of mutagenic pyrolysis products from animal acids. *Agric. Biol. Chem.,* **42,** 1235–1238.

Moutschen, J. (1960) Modifications with cystamine of chromosome damage caused by maleic hydrazide in broad bean. *Radiobiol. Lat.,* **3,** 271–277.

Moutschen, J., Moutschen-Dahmen, M., and Gillet, C. (1956) Sur les modifications induites par les hydrazides maléique et isonicotinique dans les anthéridies de *Chara vulgaris* L. *Cellule*, **58,** 65–78.

Mukherjee, R.N., and Sobels, F.H. (1968) The effects of sodium fluoride and iodoacetamide on mutation induction by X-irradiation in mature spermatozoa of *Drosophila. Mutat. Res.,* **6,** 217–225.

Novick, A. (1957) Mutagens and antimutagens. Symp. no. 8 'Mutation' *Brookhaven Symposium in Biology* (1955) (2 ed.): 201–215.

Oehlkers, F. (1953) Chromosome breaks influenced by chemicals. Symposium on chromosome breakage. *Heredity*, **6** (*Suppl.*), 95–105.

Rinkus, S.J., and Legator, M.S. (1980) The need for both *in vitro* and *in vivo* systems in mutagenicity screening. In *Chemical Mutagens* (see de Serres and Hollaender in Gen. Refs.), Vol. 6, pp. 365–473.

Röhrborn, G., and 29 participants (1978) A correlated study of cytogenic effect of isoniazid (INH) on cell systems of mammals and man conducted by thirteen laboratories. *Hum. Genet.,* **42,** 1–60.

Schmid, W. (1976) The micronucleus test for cytogenetic analysis. In *Chemical Mutagens* (see Hollaender in Gen. Refs.), Vol. 4, pp. 31–53.

Schöneich, J. (1976) Safety evaluation based on microbial assay procedures. *Mutat. Res.,* **41,** 89–94.

Schubert, J. (1969) Mutagenicity and cytotoxicity of irradiated food and food components. *Bull. WHO,* **41,** 873–904.

Schubert, J. (1972) A program to abolish harmful chemicals. *Ambio*, **3,** 79–89.

Stich, H.F., WU, C.H., and Powrie, W. (1982) Enhancement and suppression of genotoxicity of food by naturally occurring components in these products. In *Environmental Mutagens and Carcinogens* (see Sugimura, *et al.* in Gen. Refs.), pp. 347–353.

Sugimura, T. (1979) Naturally occurring genotoxic carcinogens. In Miller, J.A., Mitter, E.C., Sugimura, T., Takayama, S., and Hirono, I., *Naturally Occurring Carcinogens — Mutagens and Modulators of Carcinogenesis,* pp. 241–261.

Vogel, E. (1973) Strong antimutagenic effects of fluoride on mutation induction by Trenimon and 1-phenyl-3,3-dimethyltriazene in *Drosophila melanogaster. Mutat. Res.,* **20,**, 339–352.

Von Wettstein, D., Gustafsson, Å., and Ehrenberg, L. (1959) Mutationsforschung und Züchtung. *Arbeitsgem. Forsch. Landes Nordrhein-Westfalen,* **73,** 7–60.

Westergaard, M. (1957) Chemical mutagenesis in relation to the concept of the gene. *Experientia,* **13,** 224–234.

Zamenhof, P. (1969) On the identity of two bacterial mutator genes: effects of anti-mutagens. *Mutat. Res.,* **7,** 463–465.

Index